Succeeding in the BioMedical Admission (BMAT)

Nicola Hawley and Matt Green

develop
medica

Published by Developmedica
Castle Court
Duke Street
New Basford,
Nottingham, NG7 7JN
0115 720 0025
www.developmedica.com

Developmedica recommend that you consult the Cambridge Assessment website, Universities and Colleges Admissions Service (UCAS) and University websites for information relating to guidance on the applicability of sitting the BMAT in your application to a university in the UK. The views expressed in this book are those of Developmedica and not those of Cambridge Assessment or UCAS. Developmedica is in no way associated with Cambridge Assessment or UCAS.

The contents of this book are intended as a guide only and although every effort has been made to ensure that the contents of this book are correct, Developmedica cannot be held responsible for the outcome of any loss or damage that arises through the use of this guide. Readers are advised to seek independent advice regarding completing their BMAT together with consulting the institution the reader intends to apply to.

A catalogue record for this title is available from the British Library

ISBN 978–1–906839–00–0

Typeset by RefineCatch Limited, Bungay, Suffolk
Printed by Bell and Bain, Glasgow

Dedication

We would both like to thank Viv and Terry, for their inspiration, love and support over the years.

Other books in the Developmedica range available at www.developmedica.com

'The Developmedica Guide to Writing your Medical School Personal Statement: Your way, Successfully'

This engaging, easy to use and comprehensive book covers every aspect involved in the planning, writing and refining of your medical school Personal Statement. Aimed at school leavers, graduates and mature individuals applying to medical school, together with parents and teachers, this book will help you to write a compelling and convincing medical school Personal Statement.

'Succeeding in your Medical School Interview'

'Succeeding in your Medical School Interview' sets out the principles for success. The book highlights the importance of preparation – 'Your Homework' – and provides a framework through which you can effectively handle any question from the interview panel.

'Becoming a Doctor: Is Medicine Really the Career for You?'

Is Medicine really the career for you? Do you really want to be a Doctor? If you want answers to these questions then read Developmedica's no nonsense guide to finding out more about becoming a doctor and what a career in medicine really entails.

'Succeeding in the 2009 UK Clinical Aptitude Test (UKCAT)'

With virtually all medical school and dental schools requiring the completion of the UKCAT as part of the application process it is crucial that applicants are as fully prepared as possible. This book contains clear guidance on how to approach each section of the test, consolidates this through providing many practice questions and culminates in a full mock test that can be completed under timed conditions.

Entrance Exam, Personal Statement and Interview Support

Developmedica are committed to helping proactive candidates make successful applications to medical and dental schools in the United Kingdom. In addition to our range of books we also offer the following services:

- Personal Statement Advisory Services to help you to enhance your Personal Statement
- Entrance Exam Advice – UKCAT and BMAT practice papers and revision courses
- 'Writing Your Personal Statement, Your Way' – a one day course which takes you step by step through how to formulate your Personal Statement
- 'Medical' or 'Dental School Interview Workshops' – one day courses which will help to fully prepare you for your approaching interview and includes a mock interview
- We also offer 'Personal Statement' and 'University Interview' workshops direct to schools and colleges

For more information regarding all of our services please visit our website or call us on our freephone number:

www.developmedica.com

0115 720 0025

Testimonials

Below are what some of the readers have thought of 'Succeeding in the 2009 Biomedical Admissions Test (BMAT)':

'I found this book really helpful in helping me to know what I would be faced with in my BMAT test'
BD, Norwich

'Excellent resource – highly recommended'
LG, London'

'Having received very little guidance from my school on how to prepare for the BMAT this book was a lifesaver!'
PD, Nottingham

'What can I say! My score was one of the highest in my school and all thanks to you!'
LT, Bristol

'I have just completed my BMAT and am pleased to say that having used your book I found the test much less trouble than I thought I would'
GG, Manchester

'One word – Thank-you'
HS, Reading

'After debating whether or not to avoid medical schools requiring the BMAT your book gave me the confidence to go for it which I don't think I would have done otherwise'
PL, Southampton

Contents

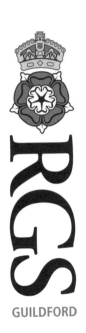

About the Authors

Nicola Hawley, BSc (Hons)

After completing her BSc in Biochemistry at Leeds University Nicola accepted a research post within the School of Biomedical Sciences at Nottingham University. This involved working in a multidisciplinary team alongside medical professionals researching the therapeutic potential of G Protein Coupled Receptors, in particular Beta-1 and Beta-2 Adrenoreceptors. Nicola now teaches science within a secondary school environment.

Matt Green, BSc (Hons), MPhil

After completing his BSc in Biochemistry Matt went on to complete an MPhil at the Royal Marsden Hospital in London. This involved working closely with medical professionals on a number of projects developing novel drugs for the treatment of ovarian cancer. After establishing a private tuition service in 2004, Matt went on to found Developmedica in 2005, and for the last five years has been working to help prospective medical students secure their first choice University place.

Preface

This book is intended to help prospective medical and veterinary studies students prepare for their Biomedical Admissions Test (BMAT). Even though the BMAT is only a requirement for a limited number of medical and veterinary schools, it is an essential part of the assessment process for those universities and the results will have a direct impact on your likelihood of acceptance.

This book covers all three sections of the BMAT, providing suggestions on how to prepare for each section and worked examples of the types of questions you will encounter during the test.

The book also contains a full mock of the BMAT, enabling you to gain an appreciation of how you will be examined. We recommend that this test is performed under exam conditions, in order to fully prepare yourself for the real thing. To gain the full benefit of this book we recommend that you visit our website to access our BMAT book product page where you can download a free answer sheet to use when working through the mock test questions.

The information in this book should be used in conjunction with information from Cambridge Assessment (www.admissionstests.cambridgeassessment.org.uk/adt/bmat) and any guidance given to you by the institutions you intend to apply to.

Chapter 1 Introduction to the BMAT

What is the BMAT?

Everyone knows that you have to have good scientific knowledge to be a successful doctor or veterinarian, but there's more to it than just achieving good grades in your science subjects. You need to be able to demonstrate excellent problem-solving skills, the ability to reason, and the ability to use all your scientific knowledge in the right way. You also need to be able to perform under pressure, whilst expressing your arguments and ideas in a clear and concise way that others can understand; the BMAT examines all of these attributes.

The BMAT, or BioMedical Admissions Test, was designed by Cambridge Assessment to help universities to refine their admissions processes. With thousands of applications to study Medicine and Veterinary Science each year and limited places, universities needed a way to differentiate between students with similar levels of ability and suitability. The BMAT provides a way for students from all educational backgrounds, including mature and overseas students, to be assessed by using equal standards.

Whilst the BMAT will assess you on many of the skills required to be a good doctor or vet, the test will primarily assess how well you are likely to cope with the rigours of university. Research into student performance in the BMAT has shown that the tests provide a good indication of how a student will perform at undergraduate level in Medicine and Veterinary

Science. This means that the universities will place a great deal of emphasis on your results when deciding whether or not to offer you a place, so it's important to prepare yourself for the exam as much as you possibly can!

This book will explore the BMAT in detail, examining the types of questions which will be asked, suggesting ways to prepare for the exam and providing worked examples to demonstrate how to answer the questions. We will also provide sample questions for you to attempt yourself, enabling you to better understand the BMAT and what will be expected of you on the day. The ultimate aim is that you will be as prepared as you possibly can be for the exam and that you will be one step closer to achieving your goal of studying at university.

Contents of the BMAT

The BMAT is a paper-based assessment divided into three sections, each of which is designed to test specific knowledge and abilities. Unlike the GCSE and A-level exams you're already taking, the BMAT will be testing you largely on basic skills and knowledge that you should already possess, rather than your academic ability. The test will examine a variety of qualities and abilities, including your ability to read formal English and follow written instructions, using different types of question throughout each section.

You will have two hours to answer a total of 63 questions from the following sections:

Section 1: Aptitude and Skills (1 hour)

During your degree, you will often face difficult problems which require you to assess a given set of information and draw conclusions based on your logic, reasoning and under-standing of raw quantitative data.

This problem solving section will test your ability to:

- Generalise or make logical deductions based on numerical and/or graphical data
- Identify, extract and understand meanings from long or complex texts
- Read and understand simple quantitative data, in numerical or graphical form, and produce simple graphs and diagrams based on this data

It is important to note that each question in this section may test you on two or more of the above.

Section 2: Scientific Knowledge and Application (30 minutes)

The second section, which is also multiple choice, will test your ability to apply scientific knowledge to given scenarios. The questions will be drawn from GCSE level Science (up to higher-level double award) and Maths.

This section will test your ability to:

- Approach problems logically, using evidence-based reasoning
- Recall basic theoretical knowledge under pressure
- Apply your knowledge of a variety of disciplines, many of which you may not have had a great deal of exposure to.

Section 3: Writing Task (30 minutes)

As a student, and subsequently as a doctor or vet, you will encounter many statements, assumptions and concepts; you will have to be prepared to challenge these concepts, examining them from every angle to develop an understanding of not only *how* but *why* things are as they are.

This section will test your ability to:

- Communicate your knowledge, arguments and deductions through clear and concise language or diagrams
- Create rational, logical and well-rounded arguments based on medical or scientific concepts
- Adopt a critical approach and consider alternative arguments when formulating a point of view.

Later in this book we will break each section down, giving examples of how to answer each section effectively and what you need to do to prepare yourself fully.

When sitting the BMAT you will be provided with an answer sheet; for Sections 1 and 2 this will either involve circling the correct multiple choice answer(s), or writing short verbal or numerical answers directly into spaces provided. The Section 3 answer sheet is discussed later on in this book.

Examples of all three answer sheets can be found on the BMAT website at:

www.admissionstests.cambridgeassessment.org.uk/adt/ bmat/practice

How is the BMAT scored?

You will record your answers on a separate sheet that will be marked electronically. For each individual question asked in Sections 1 and 2 a total of 1 mark is available. Your marks for each section will be totaled and converted to the BMAT scale. This will give you a score between 1 (low) and 9 (high). Your score will be given to one decimal place. The majority of candidates will score approximately 5 on each section which equates to a score of approximately 50%. Stronger candidates will score 6, and only exceptional candidates 7 and above.

Your essay in Section 3 will be marked holistically and given a score between 1 (low) and 15 (high). The score you are given will reflect the overall quality of the essay, and will be awarded on a three-mark scale (0, 3, 6, 9, 12, 15).

Every essay is double marked. If the marks are similar an average of the two is reported. If the marks differ significantly the essay will be marked for a third time and a final mark given is checked by a senior member of the Cambridge Assessment staff.

Your results will be issued to you in early December. The score you are awarded is final and cannot be challenged.

Who uses the BMAT?

Currently, the BMAT is used by the following universities as part of their admissions process:

- University of Cambridge (**www.cam.ac.uk/**)
- University of Oxford (**www.ox.ac.uk/**)
- Imperial College London (**www3.imperial.ac.uk/**)
- University College London (**www.ucl.ac.uk/**)
- Royal Veterinary College (**www.rvc.ac.uk/**)

Each university uses the results of the BMAT in their own way, and will accept different scores as part of their admissions requirements – you should look at your individual course requirements to see what score your university will require.

Ultimately, each university will use the results in conjunction with your UCAS application, personal statement and interview to decide whether or not to offer you a place on its Medicine or Veterinary Science course. The more prepared you are for the BMAT, the better chance you have of winning that university place!

Currently, the BMAT is a requirement for entry on to the following courses:

University of Cambridge (C05)

- Medicine (A100)
- Graduate Course in Medicine (A100) – note that the BMAT is not essential for this course
- Veterinary Medicine (D100)

University of Oxford (O33)

- Medicine (A100)
- Physiological Sciences (B100)

Imperial College London (I50)

- Medicine (A100)
- Biomedical Science – 3 year course (B900)
- Pharmacology and Translational Medical Science (BB29)
- Pharmacology and Translational Medical Science with a year in industry (BB2X)

University College London (U80)

- Medicine (A100)

Royal Veterinary College (R84)

- Veterinary Medicine (D100)
- Combined Degree Programme (D101)

How do I arrange my BMAT?

Even though you are required to take the BMAT as part of your university application, it is ultimately your responsibility to arrange the test by the required date.

Registering for the exam

The first step is to register with a BMAT centre, as it is not possible to register yourself to take the test. If you are attending school or college, talk to your Examinations Officer about the possibility of having the test arranged on your behalf. If your school or college is unable to arrange the test or if you are not currently attending school or college, then you will need to register with an open testing centre. You can find a list of centres, together will full contact details, at:

www.admissionstests.cambridgeassessment.org.uk/adt/ bmat/registration

Exam dates

Just like your UCAS application, your registration for the BMAT must be completed by a set deadline. The important dates for entry in 2008 are:

Mid September	last date for requests for modified papers (e.g. Braille or enlarged papers)
Late September	standard closing date (standard entry fees apply until 5pm GMT)
Mid October	last date for late entries (entries are not accepted after this date, and late entry fees apply until 5pm GMT)
Early November	the date of the actual BMAT exam
Early December	results are released to candidates through the BMAT centres

Costs

Taking the BMAT does incur a small fee; the fee will depend on your status and when you apply, and you should also ensure that the centre you are registered with does not charge its own administrative fees on top of this.

Costs for 2008 BMAT entry are:

£31	standard entry for a UK candidate
£62	late entry fee for a UK candidate
£54	standard entry fee for an international candidate
£108	late entry fee for an international candidate

Students who are eligible for Education Maintenance Allowance (EMA) or equivalent funding may be eligible to apply for reimbursement of these fees.

Preparing for the BMAT

As an aptitude test, the BMAT will not be examining your ability to understand and remember complex scientific information. The universities will be able to determine your level of knowledge from your A-level results; instead, they will be looking to assess your innate intelligence and personal ability coupled with your scientific understanding at GCSE level. This means that you won't necessarily need to learn a whole lot of new information for the exam, but it also means that you can't just cram for a week and hope to get a high mark!

Although the BMAT is specifically designed to negate the need for extra revision, this doesn't mean that there aren't ways to prepare for each section of the exam. Later on in this book we will explore each section in further detail and suggest ways in which you can better prepare yourself for the types of question you will be answering at each stage.

There are techniques which will help you in each particular section, but there are also more general tips which will help you to prepare for the exam as a whole. These include:

- Reading further books on critical thinking and problem solving (see reading list at the end of this book)
- Working through old exam papers to improve your general knowledge on scientific and mathematical problems
- Keeping an eye on the news and on journals to learn about new developments or current debates in medicine
- Completing mock BMAT papers and practice questions to familiarise yourself with the exam.

Always bear in mind that the BMAT is not designed to trick you or to catch you out in any way. You are being tested on *ability* rather than *knowledge*. Although some sections do test your knowledge, you will only be questioned on topics you should already know quite well. As such there is no 'right' or 'wrong' way to approach this exam, though the hints and tips we provide throughout this book should enable you to be as prepared as possible for the exam.

Chapter 2 Succeeding in the BMAT

Practise makes perfect

As with any test it is essential to practise example questions to ensure you are familiar with the structure and type of content you will be tested on. The BMAT is no exception despite what people may tell you!

The following chapters will enable you to practise each of the different sections which together form the BMAT. Each chapter contains questions to provide you with an insight into what you will be faced with in the test, and aims to help you to put into practice what you learn. This will enable you to familiarise yourself with the format and style of the BMAT and hopefully help you to realise that most of the questions in the test will be of general ability.

However, this is not to say that the BMAT test is of an easy nature, otherwise it would not be a valid measure in the selection process. Although the BMAT may measure general ability you will find that you only have a limited amount of time for each section.

Each of the sections is individually timed, therefore it is not possible for you to make up for lost time in the other remaining sections. It is vital that you complete each section fully as you progress through the test and do not leave any questions unanswered. Unlike conventional tests you are unable to go back and finish off unanswered questions from previous sections.

It may therefore be valuable to time yourself when you undertake the mock test at the end of this book. This way you will be able to enhance your time management skills, together with increasing your confidence and also alleviate any anxiety you may have. The aim of this book is to ensure that, on the day of your test, you are faced with something you are already familiar with.

This book culminates with a full mock test for you to complete under timed conditions. An answer sheet can be downloaded for free from www.developmedica.com to help you make the most of this book.

What are multiple choice tests?

The BMAT is set out in a multiple choice or short answer format, with the exception of Section 3 which we will address later in this book. These types of tests are commonly used within the field of selection and assessment. The test questions are designed to test a candidate's awareness and understanding of a particular subject.

The sections within the BMAT are based on an answer format known as 'A Type Questions', which is the most commonly used design in multiple choice tests. This specific design helps to make transparent the number of choices which need to be selected. These questions usually consist of a 'Stem and Lead-in Question' which is followed by a 'series' of 'choices', or a request for a short numerical or verbal answer. To illustrate this, below is an example of a question you may be faced with:

Stem

This is generally an introductory statement, question or passage of relevant information which elicits the correct answer. The stem on the whole provides all the information for the question or questions which will follow e.g.

'There are 100 students who go on a school trip to a science park.'

Lead-in Question

This is the question which identifies the exact answer e.g.

'35% of the students were female, how many female students were there?'

Choices

In a multiple choice test, the choices will generally consist of one correct answer. However, depending on the type of question, you may be required to find two or even three correct answers. Wherever there are correct answers there are also incorrect answers, which are also known as the 'distracters'. For the above example, typical choices could be as follows:

A. *25*
B. *67*
C. *35 – Correct answer (35% of 100 students = 35 female students)*
D. *65*

Alternatively you may simply be asked to state the number in the space provided.

Tips for Succeeding in the BMAT

- To help you with your time management ensure you take a watch or timer with you to the test.
- Read, and **re-read the question** to ensure you fully understand what is being asked, not what you want to be asked
- **Eliminate any incorrect answers** you know are incorrect
- Read the question and try to answer it before looking at the choices available to you
- Ensure you record your answers clearly as Sections 1 and 2 are marked by computers
- When you enter a written answer (particularly in Section 3) ensure you write clearly and legibly
- Ensure when changing your answers you erase the old answer thoroughly
- **Do not spend too much time on one question** – remember you only have a set amount of time per section so, as a rule of thumb, you should spend x amount per question (x = time of section ÷ number of questions)
- **Do not keep changing your mind** – research has shown that the 1st answer that appeals to you is often the correct one
- If you cannot decide between two answers – look carefully and decide whether for one of the options you are making an unnecessary assumption – **trust your gut instinct**
- Always select an answer for a given question even if you do not know the answer – **never leave any answers blank**

- **Pace yourself** – you will need to work through the test at the right speed. Too fast and your accuracy may suffer, too slow and you may run out of time. Use this book to practise your time keeping and approach to answering each question – you need to do what works for you, not what might work for someone else

- Try to leave some time at the end of each section to check your answers.

- To familiarise yourself with the way the test will be conducted visit the BMAT website which also contains further practice tests

- Remember you will only be awarded marks for correct answers, and marks will not be deducted for incorrect answers. Therefore **answer every single question**, even ones you are unsure of

- When you take the test, listen carefully to the administrator's instructions

- If you are unsure about anything, remember to ask the test administrator before the test begins. Once the clock begins ticking, interruptions will not be allowed

- You may be presented with a question which you simply cannot answer due to difficulty or if the wording is too vague. If you have only approximately 90 seconds per question, and you find yourself spending five minutes determining the answer for each question then your time management skills are poor and you are wasting valuable time

- Do not be alarmed if the test is different from the practice papers you have worked through, remember you are being tested primarily on aptitude

Chapter 3 Section 1: Aptitude and Skills

Overview of Section 1

Problem-solving skills are essential for any medical or veterinary student; you will often be called upon to resolve problems arising from complex ideas or concepts, most likely under pressure, and will have to call on your powers of logical and analytical thinking to succeed. The practice of evidence-based medicine is a current issue of debate in the medical profession and being able to make judgements based on limited data is a difficult technique to perfect. As a doctor, this skill will be vital in making on-the-spot decisions, many of which could be life-or-death, based on the evidence presented to you.

Section 1 will test your ability to analyse and reason through various mathematical, logical and observational scenarios. You will have a total of **1 hour** to complete 35 multiple-choice questions. You will be provided with an answer sheet, where you will circle the correct multiple-choice answer(s), or write short verbal or numerical answers directly into the spaces provided. One very important thing to remember is that you are **not** allowed to use a calculator for this section, so all working out must be done on the exam paper itself or in your head.

A maximum of 35 marks are available in this section.

Section 1 is divided into three further sub-sections:

- Problem solving (30 mins)
- Understanding arguments (15 mins)
- Data analysis and inference (15 mins)

Each sub-section will test you using different types of questions (these are covered in the individual sections of the chapter). The common theme of the questions will be that you will be presented with a set of data – numerical, textual or graphical – and will be asked to come to a conclusion based entirely on the evidence presented to you. If a question is multiple choice, you will have to narrow down your answer choices to find the answer (or answers if the question asks for more than one) which best fits the question. Eliminating incorrect answers first can help you to identify the correct answer.

Note that the sections will not appear in the exact order above, but will appear randomly from each sub-section. The timings are to give an idea of what proportion of Section 1 will be taken up by each sub-section, and thus roughly how long you should be taking on each type of question. It is also important to note that a question may assess you on two or more of the above skills.

The next few sections will explore how you can prepare for Section 1, and will work through some examples to allow you to get to grips with the kinds of questions you will be answering.

Preparing for Section 1

As this section involves purely 'evidence-based' questions, there are no subjects to revise beforehand. Whilst this may make preparation sound more difficult, there are ways in which you can prepare for Section 1.

This section will test you on your ability to:

- Address the type of complex problems you could be faced with in your future career
- Interpret scientific data and concepts
- Draw conclusions from arguments and information presented to you

Section 1 focuses on technique, not knowledge; the best way to succeed is to focus on *how* to answer the questions. The most obvious way to do this – practice! Spend as much time as you can working through example questions and papers so that you know exactly what will be asked of you in the exam. Whenever possible, practise under timed conditions; there's no point in knowing how to answer the questions if you can't do it in the allotted time, so find a quiet space, set your stopwatch and see how well you can do. Each time you practise, you should get better at answering the questions within the required time.

You could also spend some time reading up on problem-solving or analytical techniques. This isn't essential, and won't provide the same benefits as practising the questions directly, but it might give you ideas on how to spot the correct answers or how to improve your timing. Be careful though, as many of these books will probably be more in-depth than you need, and may explore skills that aren't completely relevant to the BMAT.

Sub-section: Problem Solving

This sub-section will include both numerical and logical problems (equivalent of Key Stage 4 curriculum), designed to assess your ability to think a situation through logically and precisely. You will need to look at the information provided and work systematically towards the answer by first establishing all of the possibilities, then eliminating them one by one until you reach your answer. Some of the skills required for this sub-section are:

- Identifying the appropriate (and inappropriate) data in the information provided to enable you to answer the question – an important skill required of medical professionals
- Recognising patterns and trends within data and reapplying this information to new data sets
- Selecting the correct approach or formula to determine the correct answer from the information provided, often combing multiple data sets – always read the question in its entirety to ensure that you identify the bigger picture

In the following pages we will examine the types of questions you will encounter in the problem solving sub-section.

Example Question 1

Five friends are queuing up together for tickets to their favourite band. Darren is behind Andy, who is behind Brian. Edward is in front of Chris, but behind Andy.

Chris must be:

A   Behind Brian and ahead of Darren

B   Behind Andy, but not necessarily behind Darren

C   Behind Darren and ahead of Edward

D   Ahead of Brian, but not necessarily behind Andy

Answer

These questions are fairly self-explanatory, but don't be caught out by trying to work it out in your head. The best way to work through this is to draw it all out and work through it visually. This is where the blank pages in the exam paper come in useful! Based on what we're given above, there are a number of constants: no-one is ahead of Brian; Andy is behind Brian; and Chris, Darren and Edward are behind Andy. This leads to three possibilities:

Brian, Andy, Edward, **Chris**, Darren

Brian, Andy, Darren, Edward, **Chris**

Brian, Andy, Edward, Darren, **Chris**

Now it's just a process of elimination. At no point could Chris be ahead of Edward, so that rules out Option C. He also cannot be ahead of Brian, which rules out Option D. He is definitely behind Brian, but even though he is likely to be behind Darren, this isn't definite which rules out Option A. The most likely answer, then, is **Option B**.

Example Question 2

If someone suffers a migraine, they will experience a painful headache. Most, though not all, sufferers of migraines may also suffer from nausea, flashing lights, sickness, and sensitivity to light and sound.

Based on the information above, which option, from A to F, correctly places the following sentences in order of probability, with the most probable first?

1. Anyone suffering from a migraine will experience nausea and sensitivity to light and sound
2. Anyone experiencing a migraine will experience a headache or sickness

3. Anyone suffering from a migraine will experience a headache, possibly accompanied by flashing lights and sickness

A   3, 2, 1
B   2, 3, 1
C   1, 2, 3
D   2, 1, 3
E   3, 1, 2
F   1, 3, 2

Answer:

Let's examine this question in a little more detail. First, the question itself:

If someone suffers a migraine, they will experience a painful headache. Most, though not all, sufferers of migraines may also suffer from nausea, flashing lights, sickness, and sensitivity to light and sound.

The passage is formed of two separate sentences. The first is a definite, signified by 'will'. The second is more conditional, signified by 'may'. This is the first step to answering this question – differentiating between what '*will*' and what '*could*' happen. It's vital to remember that your answer should be based on the evidence presented in the question, not on what you may already know about the subject. You may be a migraine sufferer and you may always experience a headache and nausea together, but that information isn't relevant to the question. Only use what's right in front of you, even if you think it is factually incorrect.

The second part of the question is telling you what you are required to do:

Which option, from A to F, correctly places the following sentence in order of probability, with the most probable first?

In this case, you are being asked to look at options A to F and determine which one best describes the order of the three following sentences. Pay particular attention to that last part of the question; the option you are looking for should place the *most* probable *first*. This will not always be the case, and some questions may ask you to place the *least* probable first. Make sure you read the question fully and understand what's being asked of you.

Let's look at the three sentences and determine the probabilities of each one:

1. *Anyone suffering from a migraine will experience nausea and sensitivity to light and sound*

The first point of note is that this is a definite statement ('will'). Looking back at the question, we are told that 'most' migraine sufferers will experience nausea and sensitivity to light. The only definite symptom of a migraine is a headache, so this option doesn't seem entirely probable.

2. *Anyone experiencing a migraine will experience a headache or sickness*

Like the first statement, this statement has a definite element ('will'). However, there is also a conditional element ('or'). Consider the alternatives of the 'or' element; according to the information provided, a migraine could consist of a headache alone, but it could not consist of sickness alone. As such, this statement is either highly probable or highly improbable. However, because the statement includes an 'or' and not an 'and', this statement still carries a higher probability than statement 1.

3. *Anyone suffering from a migraine will experience a headache, possibly accompanied by flashing lights and sickness*

Again, we have a definite element ('will'), but we also have a conditional element ('possibly accompanied' acts as a 'may'). The first part we can deduce to be correct, as we can deduce that a headache is a definite symptom of a migraine. However, we can also deduce that flashing lights and sickness are also possible accompanying symptoms. This is where we must decide on where this statement fits in terms of probabilities; the probability of having a headache *and* accompanying symptoms is higher than that of having a headache *or* other symptoms, so statement 3 is more probable than statement 2.

Based on the above arguments, the answer is Option **A**: 3, 2, 1 as the most likely order of statements.

Example Question 3

A plumber charges a flat rate call out charge and an hourly rate for every job he does. In one day he does two jobs, one for four hours which earns him £73, and one for five and a half hours which earns him £91.

Calculate:

i)   His call out charge
ii) His hourly rate

Answer

The first thing to do is to express his earnings as an equation, where x can be his hourly rate and y his flat call out charge.

So for his first job: $4x + y = 73$ (Equation 1)
And his second: $5.5x + y = 91$ (Equation 2)
If we rearrange Equation 1 we can make y the subject:

$4x + y = 73$
$y = 73 - 4x$

We can now substitute y into Equation 2.

$5.5x + y = 91$
$5.5x + (73 - 4x) = 91$
$1.5x + 73 = 91$
$1.5x = 18$
$x = £12$

We now substitute the value of x into Equation 1:

$4(12) + y = 73$
$48 + y = 73$
$y = 73 - 48$
$y = £25$

So his call out charge is £25, and his hourly rate £12.

Sub-section: Understanding Arguments

This sub-section will use short passages of text, usually just a paragraph, or small data sets, to test your ability to quickly identify and understand arguments. There are many ways in which these questions can be phrased, but the core principle behind each question will be the same: assess a given set of information and, using your skills of reasoning, work towards the answer you are asked to find. This may be multiple choice or may request a short written or numerical answer. It is vital you only use the information you are given, and not your prior knowledge.

The main skills this sub-section will evaluate you on are:

- Inference – determining reliable conclusions from the information provided and, where applicable, identifying unsafe ones
- Ability to analyse – determining the motivations, themes, assumptions and any conclusions in a given set of information
- Effectively evaluating information – determining flaws and errors in given information, identifying pros and cons in an argument and whether the information supports these arguments.

Questions may ask for the following information:

- What is the main conclusion of the information provided?
- Which of the below indicates a flaw in the passage above?
- Which of the below options would further strengthen the above conclusion?
- What is the main assumption of the argument presented in the passage?

It is important to have a clear understanding of the definition of some of the terms used in these question types:

- Conclusion: a proposition concluded or inferred from the premises of an argument
- Assumption: something taken for granted
- Explanation: something that explains; a statement made to clarify something and make it understandable
- Inference: derived by reasoning; conclusions or judgements made/based on premises or evidence

- Implication: the relationship between two propositions, or classes of propositions, by virtue of which one is logically deducible from the other
- Flaw: indication that a given meaning results in an argument or conclusion being unjust
- Justification: a reason, fact, circumstance, or explanation that justifies or defends
- Reason: a statement presented in justification or explanation of a belief or action
- Ambiguous: of doubtful or uncertain nature; difficult to comprehend, distinguish, or classify
- Anomaly: an odd, peculiar, or strange condition, situation or quality
- Discrepancy: an instance of difference or inconsistency
- Definition: the act of defining or making definite, distinct, or clear.

Succeeding in the Understanding Arguments Sub-section

- Ensure the answer you give is determined solely on the information contained within the passage.
- Look out for misleading words such as '*all*', '*everything*' and '*completely*' – these are specific types of words which suggest that the whole of a particular object, person, area or group are wholly affected.
- Other misleading words include 'virtually', 'almost', 'particularly', 'nearly' and 'close to' – these are words which refer to something *close to* happening rather than actually happening.
- It is very important that you read the passages very carefully.

One common mistake that candidates often make is to allow their previous knowledge on a subject to interfere with and bias the information and facts that are presented in the passages (often these are of a conflicting nature).

- Remember that each of the passages is deliberately manipulated to influence the candidate to a particular perspective or point of view.

- Often you may find that a passage states information which may subsequently alter or be contradicted further on in the passage. Ensure that you note any changes or contradictions and reflect these when selecting your answers.

- Do not waste too much time thinking about a difficult question. All questions are marked equally, therefore a difficult question will not be worth more than an easy question and vice versa. If you are having difficulty understanding a passage, flag it and move on to the next passage and come back to it later.

- Remember time management is key throughout the test.

- If you find a question particularly difficult you can flag it so that you can return to it before you move onto the next subtest.

- Attempt all questions as you will not be penalised for getting questions wrong, but you will lose marks if you leave any answers blank.

- Learn to manage your time efficiently. Go through practice mock papers and time yourself as if you were in a real exam. By familiarising yourself with the types of questions you will be faced with you will be able to analyse where your weaknesses are and improve.

- Read through newspapers and various other sources of literature which use elaborate and detailed language. This will enhance your skills in reading and also enable you to consider in-depth critical arguments and perspectives.

The following example questions cover some of the types of questions you will be asked, though this is by no means an exhaustive list.

Example Question 1

Diabetes can be caused by a number of factors. The most common form of diabetes, Type 2, is frequently linked with obesity, and exercise and healthy eating are often prescribed as a means of management. Ageing can also be a factor, and a family history of diabetes increases the risk of developing the condition. The combination of causing factors can make it extremely difficult to predict the emergence and severity of Type 2 diabetes.

Which one of the following statements best summarises the above information?

A   It is not possible to predict Type 2 diabetes in people
B   A healthy lifestyle will help prevent you from developing diabetes
C   Diabetes can be caused by eating lots of sugary food
D   Young, slim people are unlikely to suffer from diabetes
E   Obesity is a significant, though not the only, factor affecting diabetes

Answer:

These types of question often appear to be much more difficult than they are. As you only have a short time to complete the questions in, the idea of reading passages of text may be daunting, but don't forget that the questions are designed to be relatively straightforward. Once you've looked at the information presented to you, let's look at what we're being asked to do:

Which one of the following statements best summarises the above information?

Make sure you read this carefully; this question is asking you to pick the *one* statement that best summarises the passage. You may be asked to pick more than one statement, so make sure you do what the question is asking.

The best approach to these types of question is to quickly determine and eliminate which of the answers is definitely incorrect. Work your way down to the most likely answers and then compare them to see which one looks the most accurate. Let's look through each of the statements and see which ones best fit the information we've been given:

A　　*It is not possible to predict Type 2 diabetes in people*

The last line of the passage states that it is 'extremely difficult to predict the emergence and severity of Type 2 diabetes', rather than impossible. This statement is, therefore, not a good summary.

B　　*A healthy lifestyle will help prevent you from developing diabetes*

This is certainly suggested, as it is stated that 'exercise and healthy eating are often prescribed as a means of management'. However, this is only a passing mention.

C　　*Diabetes can be caused by eating lots of sugary food*

Obesity is put forward as a potential cause of diabetes; you may know that eating lots of sugary food can cause obesity, but that isn't mentioned in the passage. Based on the information given to us, this isn't a good summary.

D   *Young, slim people are unlikely to suffer from diabetes*

This certainly fits the information given to us; we are told that obesity and age are factors in diabetes, but does this summarise the passage as a whole?

E   *Obesity is a significant, though not the only, factor affecting diabetes*

Both the first and the last sentences of the paragraph refer to the variety of causes of diabetes. We are told that obesity is a frequently suspected culprit, though ageing and genetics also play a part, so this statement would seem to be the best summary of the passage.

Based on the information given to us, we can deduce that the most likely answer is **E**.

Example Question 2

As a response to rising levels of antisocial behaviour, the government introduced the Antisocial Behaviour Order (ASBO) in 1998. ASBOs target socially disruptive behaviour, and are issued for a variety of offences including vandalism and harassment. However, ASBOs have received criticism for being too 'open-ended' and for becoming 'badges of honour' for many younger criminals.

What is the underlying assumption of this passage?

A   Only younger criminals receive ASBOs
B   Antisocial behaviour is disruptive
C   ASBOs will reduce levels of antisocial behaviour
D   Antisocial behaviour is becoming more frequent
E   ASBOs are ineffective at stopping antisocial behaviour

These questions demonstrate why it's important to read and understand what's being asked of you. Unlike the 'summarising the passage' question, you are being asked to highlight the *assumption* that is being made at the heart of the passage. The answer won't necessarily be based on anything factual in the passage, but will be something that is inferred throughout and that ultimately affects whether the information in the passage makes sense.

As with other similar questions, read the passage carefully and examine each potential assumption at a time. Eliminate the obviously incorrect answers, and then work through what is left to make a decision.

A   *Only younger criminals receive ASBOs*

It is mentioned in the passage that younger criminals often view ASBOs as 'badges of honour', but there does not appear to be any kind of indication that younger criminals are specifically targeted for ASBOs. As such, this isn't an underlying assumption of the text.

B   *Antisocial behaviour is disruptive*

We're told in the first sentence that ASBOs were introduced as a response to levels of antisocial behaviour. In the second sentence we are told that ASBOs target 'disruptive behaviour'. From this we can infer that antisocial behaviour is disruptive, and whilst this is in itself an assumption, it is not the main assumption underlying the passage.

C   *ASBOs will reduce levels of antisocial behaviour*

Again, the first sentence tells us that ASBOs were introduced because of rising levels of antisocial behaviour. We are also told that ASBOs are targeted towards disruptive behaviour. We are never told specifically that ASBOs *will* affect levels of antisocial behaviour, but as we are told that they are a response to increasing antisocial behaviour, we must assume that they are working (or why else would we use them?). This seems to be a very likely answer, but remember to look through the rest of the options before deciding.

D   *Antisocial behaviour is becoming more frequent*

This is basically a re-wording of the first sentence; as such, it's not really an assumption and can be quickly disregarded.

E   *ASBOs are ineffective at stopping antisocial behaviour*

Although we can assume that ASBOs will have an effect on antisocial behaviour, as that is what they are designed to do, there is no insinuation that they are *not* effective. The final sentence does detail criticisms of ASBOs, but does not suggest or insinuate that they are ineffective in any way.

Having looked through the possibilities, the most likely answer is **C**.

Example Question 3

Consumer Price Index (CPI) annual inflation – the Government's target measure – was 2.1% in November and in the previous month. The main increase came from the changes in the price of fuel. The average price of petrol increased by 3.5 pence per litre in November, to a standstill at £1.00 per litre. When compared to last year's prices there was an overall fall from last November of 0.2 pence per litre.

Gas and electricity bills remained constant with an average bill escalating up to almost £600 a quarter for both types of bills. The prices of the bills remained constant up until November when prices increased by 10.8%.

Which of the following statements are flawed based on the above passage:

A   In the 11th month of the year CPI annual inflation was 2.1% and the price of a litre of petrol was 100 pence

B   There was an overall fall of 0.2% compared to last year's fuel prices

C   Gas and electricity prices rose by 10.8% in November.

D   The main reason CPI annual inflation rose was due to increase in the price of fuel

Answer

Option A is correctly summed up by the first paragraph

Option B is incorrect as the fall in fuel prices is actually 0.2 pence not 0.2%

Option C is correctly summed up in the second paragraph

Option D is correctly indicated in the first paragraph

Option B is therefore the correct answer

Example Question 4

House Price Index (HPI) inflation rose to 6.7% in December, up from around 3.2% in October. The major causes which influence HPI were comparable to those affecting the CPI. However, there were additional major contributions from food and motor vehicle purchase costs and a moderately descending role from vehicle insurance.

What is the difference in HPI inflation between October and December?

A   3.5%
B   3.0%
C   3.2%
D   5.5%

Answer

A simple subtraction is required

Inflation rate in December − inflation rate in October

$= 6.7\% - 3.2\%$

$= 3.5\%$

Therefore the correct answer is A: 3.5%

Sub-section: Data Analysis and Inference

This sub-section will test your ability to analyse statistical data and select which statements best describe what the data is telling you. The questions will take the form of graphs and tables or verbal information, where you will need to first understand the data presented to you before choosing the most accurate interpretation.

For each set of data and information presented approximately four questions will be asked relating to that data. Together with some of the skills required for the Problem Solving and Understanding Arguments sub-sections you will also be required to:

- Determine conclusions from the information provided
- Manipulate further the data presented to you to deduce answers
- Interpret complex data to determine reasons for patterns or flaws

Example Question 1

Questions 1, 2 and 3 refer to the data in the table below.

The table below shows the average house prices for regions in the UK from 2005 until 2008.

	Average price (£)			
Region	2008	2007	2006	2005
North East	133,500	131,000	125,500	118,000
South East	231,500	220,000	200,000	194,500
London	360,000	350,000	300,000	279,500
East	182,500	178,500	175,000	168,500
South West	197,000	195,000	180,000	170,000
Wales	140,000	135,000	130,000	125,000
West Midlands	154,500	152,000	147,500	139,000
Yorkshire & The Humber	145,500	148,500	138,000	128,000
North West	139,000	136,000	128,000	120,500
East Midlands	143,000	145,500	138,000	133,000
National average	184,000	178,000	171,000	160,000

Which region saw the greatest percentage increase in price between the years 2006 and 2007?

A   London
B   South East
C   Wales
D   East
E   South West

Answer

Instead of wasting time calculating the price increases for all the regions, you need only calculate them for the options you are given above, as one of these must be the right answer.

For each we work out the difference in price between 2006 and 2007, which we do simply by subtracting 2006 values from those of 2007.

We then calculate the difference as a percentage increase of 2006 figures.

e.g. for London:

Price increase from 2006 to 2007 was £350,000 − £300,000 = £50,000

We then express this increase as a fraction of 2006 values:

£50,000/£300,000 = 1/6 increase

As you are not allowed a calculator it's easier and quicker to leave the difference as a fraction.

We then repeat this for the other regions:

Region	2007	2006	increase (£)	increase as a fraction
South East	220,000	200,000	20,000	1/10
London	350,000	300,000	50,000	1/6
East	178,500	175,000	3,500	1/50
South West	195,000	180,000	15,000	1/12
Wales	135,000	130,000	5,000	1/26

So the region with the biggest increase is London, Answer A.

Example Question 2

A couple bought a house in Wales in 2005 for £200,000. In 2008 they wanted to sell the house.

If the house value increases as the regional average did, how much should they expect to get for their house?

A   £224,000
B   £220,000
C   £215,000
D   £237,000
E   £210,000

Answer

First we need to calculate the average increase in house prices from 2005 to 2008 in Wales.

£140,000 − £125,000 = £15,000

We then calculate the increase as a fraction:

15,000 ÷ 125,000 = 15/125 which can be reduced to 3/25

The couple paid £200,000, so we need to calculate 3/25 of this and add it to the value.

We first calculate 1/25 of the value

£200 ÷ 25 = 8
£200,000 ÷ 25 = £8000
3/25 = £8000 × 3 = £24,000
£24,000 + £200,000 = £224,000

So the correct answer is A.

Example Question 3

What is the difference in the value of the house in 2008 if the house value was estimated using the national average instead of the regional average?

A   £24,000 more
B   £6,000 more
C   £9,000 more
D   £6,000 less
E   £9,000 less

Answer

We have already worked out the estimated value of the house using the regional averages in Wales. We need to do the same for the national average:

£184,000 − £160,000 = £24,000

We then calculate the percentage increase:

24,000 ÷ 160,000 = 24/160 which can be reduced to 3/20

The couple paid £200,000. We need to calculate 3/20 of this and add it to the value.

1/10 of £200,000 = £20,000
1/20 of £200,000 = £10,000
3/20 of £200,000 = £30,000

£30,000 + £200,000 = £230,000

We then calculate the difference between the two estimates:

£230,000 − £224, 000 = £6,000

If the property were valued using the national average it would be worth £6,000 more than if it was valued using the regional average. The answer is B.

Example Question 4

Questions 4, 5 and 6 refer to the graph below:

The graph below shows the effect of an increasing carbon dioxide concentration on breathing.

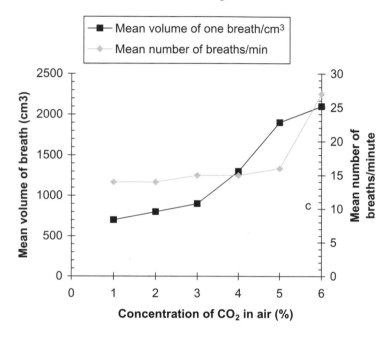

What was the average volume of air breathed in one minute at a concentration of 2% CO_2?

A   800cm³

B   11,200 cm³

C   700 cm³

D   12,000 cm³

Answer

The question asks what volume of air was breathed in a minute. We can determine from the graph that at 2% CO_2 a mean volume of 800 cm^3 is taken in per breath. The graph also tells us that at 2% CO_2 a mean of 14 breaths are performed per minute. So to calculate how much air is breathed in a minute we need to multiply the volume of air taken in on one breath by the number of breaths taken in a minute.

$= 14 \times 800$

$= 11,200$ cm^3 per minute

Therefore the correct answer is B.

Example Question 5

Between which concentrations of CO_2 is the greatest increase in the total volume of air breathed in per minute seen?

A   2–3% CO_2
B   3–4% CO_2
C   4–5% CO_2
D   5–6% CO_2

This question is similar to the one above. A common mistake to make is to look at the graph and assume the greatest increase is between 4 and 5% CO_2, where the gradient of the mean volume of one breath is greatest. However, the question asks for greatest increase in the total air breathed in per minute – so we also need to take the number of breaths per minute into consideration.

It is reasonable to say that the greatest increase is either going to be between 4–5% CO_2 or 5–6% CO_2, as we can see from the graph that the mean volume of one breath does not increase a great deal between 1 and 3% CO_2 nor does the number of breaths per minute (when compared to the increase seen at concentrations of 4% and above), so this eliminates option A.

So we can calculate the volume of air breathed in per minute for 4%, 5% and 6% CO_2 by multiplying the number of breaths in a minute by the average volume of each breath, and then calculate the differences:

4% CO_2 = 1,300 × 15 = 19,500cm^3
5% CO_2 = 1,900 × 16 = 30,400cm^3
6% CO_2 = 2,100 × 27 = 56,700cm^3

Differences between 4% and 5% = 30,400−19,500 = 10,900cm^3
Differences between 5% and 6% = 56,700−30,400 = 26,300cm^3

The greatest increase is seen between 5 and 6% CO_2.

Therefore, the correct answer is D.

Example Question 6

At a concentration of 7% CO_2 (data not shown), the mean volume of one breath was 15% greater than that at 6% CO_2. What was the mean volume of one breath at 7% CO_2?

A   2,415 cm^3
B   2,115 cm^3
C   2,205 cm^3
D   1,785 cm^3

Answer

This is just a simple percentage calculation. At 6% CO_2 2,100 cm^3 of air was breathed in each breath. So at 7% CO_2 2,100 + 15% was breathed in.

$2,100 \div 10 = 210$

So $10\% = 210$

$5\% = 210 \div 2 = 105$

So $15\% = 210 + 105 = 315$

We then add this to $2,100$ to give a 15% increase $= 2,100 + 315 = 2,415 cm^3$

A is the correct answer.

Example Question 7

Example Questions 7 to 10 refer to the following passage

The health of an individual is significantly influenced by the environment around them and the state of Planet Earth's health is often considered to be one of the largest worries facing the health of the human race in modern times. The distressed callings of what used to be considered 'ranting on a soap box' are no longer discounted by the masses and the relationship between adverse climate change and someone's health is clearly demonstrated by leading authorities such as the World Health Organisation.

The increased incidence of disease causing entities, the lack of safe drinking water, susceptibility to serious flooding and the constantly reducing number of durable crops which provide staple foods are having an impact on a global scale.

Virtually all of the countries that are most susceptible to the above risks do not have the resources and infrastructure to effectively address these hazards, whilst at the same time First World countries have been lethargic in offering their support to those that need it.

Another factor contributing to such a slow response from developed countries to provide assistance is the fact that the above incidences occur on a global scale and in such large numbers. Encouraging those that can make a difference to face up to their responsibilities is no mean feat and requires commitment to change both from a personal perspective and a government one. Future health professionals are one community that can make a positive difference to the state of the World's health in the form of both acting as role models who lead carbon neutral lifestyles and canvassing positive action in the name of improving the health of the planet.

A recent newspaper article raised the need for medical professionals to endeavour to determine the ideal average amount of carbon an individual should produce if mankind is to stand any chance of reducing and ultimately preventing 'catastrophic effects' on the planet. Based on the premise that each person must have an equal annual 'personal carbon allowance', this can be calculated at 1 tonne of carbon per person per year. A circulated questionnaire amongst medical professionals canvassing carbon usage determined a large proportion of the medical professionals created carbon emissions significantly more than 1 tonne per year. The general consensus was that the above average figure was unobtainable, which prompts the call for more proactive and creative approaches to tackling the health of the planet. 33 per cent of the UK's carbon emissions are created by the production of domestic energy production and a further 26 per cent is attributable to transport emissions. This therefore suggests that there is huge potential for reducing these emissions through relatively small changes to our everyday lives.

Initiatives such as utilising public transport, ensuring domestic appliances are switched off when not in use, or avoiding air travel through opting to spend holidays at home would have a notable effect.

Identifying and taking responsibility for the impact that mankind has on the environment and formulating positive steps to counter this is becoming increasingly important and is the only way that the World's health will begin to noticeably improve.

Question 7

If the UK's total annual carbon emissions are 300,000,000 million tonnes, how many tonnes of carbon emissions are produced by the production of domestic energy?

Answer

The passage tells us that 33% of the UK's carbon emissions is created by the production of domestic energy. If the total emissions for the UK is 300,000,000 million we simply need to calculate 33% of this.

33% of 300,000,000 million
1% = 300,000,000 million ÷ 100 = 3,000,000 million
33% = 3,000,000 million × 33 = 99,000,000 million tonnes

Question 8

Which statement is correctly inferred by the passage:

A   Initiatives such as recycling and lower emission cars are having a notable effect on reducing global warming

B   The susceptibility of countries to natural hazards is caused primarily by a lack of money

C   The effects of natural hazards on developing countries have been exacerbated by the slow response of First World countries in providing support

D   Reducing carbon emissions will not make much difference to the health of the planet

Answer

Option A is not inferred by the passage as it refers to utilising public transport, ensuring domestic appliances are switched off when not in use or avoiding air travel through opting to spend holidays at home.

Option B is not inferred by the passage as it refers to countries being susceptible to risks due to lack of resources and infrastructure to effectively address these hazards.

Option C is inferred by the passage as it states 'whilst at the same time First World countries have been lethargic in offering their support to those that need it.'

Option D is not inferred by the passage as in the final paragraph it states that formulating positive steps is the only way the World's health will begin to noticeably improve.

The correct answer is therefore Option C.

Question 9

In what entity was the article relating to medical professionals published?

A   Magazine
B   Website article
C   Newspaper
D   Tabloid

Answer

The correct answer is therefore Option C: Newspaper

Question 10

Which one or more of the options below will have a positive effect on reducing carbon emissions?

A   Ensuring domestic appliances are switched off
B   Avoiding public transport
C   Utilising air travel
D   Implementing recycling measures

Answer

The correct answer is Option A as this is stated in the penultimate paragraph.

Top tips for succeeding in Section 1

- Refresh your memory by working through your GCSE maths books to ensure you are familiar with the following:

  ➢ Addition and subtraction

  ➢ Multiplication and division

  ➢ Fractions and percentages

  ➢ Converting fractions, decimals and percentages

  ➢ Determining mode, mean and median averages

  ➢ Algebra

  ➢ Decimals

  ➢ Distance, time and speed triangles

  ➢ Calculating area and perimeters

  ➢ Analysing charts, bar charts, pie charts, frequency tables etc.

  ➢ Square and cubed numbers

- **Work through the questions systematically.** You may find that a question refers to your previous answer(s).
- **Work out all your calculations on the note paper provided.** If there are errors you may be able to determine from your rough workings at what point you made a mistake.
- Go through the practice mock papers and **identify your strengths and weaknesses early so you can improve on your weaknesses.** For example, you may be better at completing algebra equations rather than fractions.
- When answering questions which involve 'humans', remember to calculate your final answer to the nearest whole number as people cannot be represented as a decimal or a fraction! This may be an important point to take note of when converting percentages to actual numbers.
- One major pitfall is to select an option which you think is nearest to the answer. Often you will find that the majority of the options are very close to each other and may differ in terms of decimal points or a single digit which is either added or removed. Therefore it is very important to evaluate the answer options very carefully.
- Always answer questions in the correct metric units. For example, a question may ask you to calculate something in centimetres but then give your final answer in metres. Therefore it is important to **read each item very closely.**
- Some algebra questions may require you to calculate the value of 'x'. Often this will be x on its own or

sometimes the answer may require you to find x^3 or x^2. Therefore it is always important to **look at how the questions require you to give your final answer.**

- Remember to **time yourself as you complete the mock test.** This will improve your time management skills, ensuring you have adequate time to answer every question.

- If you really are unsure about a question eliminate the obvious wrong answers and then make a calculated guess. You will not be penalised for getting an answer wrong. A guess means that you have a 25 per cent chance of getting the mark, so it is better to guess than to leave the question blank!

Chapter 4 Section 2: Scientific Knowledge and Applications

Overview of Section 2

Although your A-level results will give your universities the best indication of your level of knowledge, they do not show how good you are at *using* that knowledge in the right way. Being able to remember and recite scientific or mathematical facts under exam conditions isn't enough to succeed as a doctor. Being able to apply your knowledge, including knowledge that you may not have accessed or revisited in a long time, is key to passing your Medical or Veterinary degree and becoming a skilled and knowledgeable doctor or vet.

Section 2 of the BMAT will examine your ability to apply relatively basic scientific and mathematical knowledge to given scenarios. You will have **30 minutes** to answer 27 questions on subjects drawn from GCSE Double Science (including Biology, Chemistry and Physics) and Mathematics. The difficulty of the questions will be anywhere up to higher level. Each question is worth one mark and you should expect to see between 6–8 Biology questions, 6–8 Chemistry questions, 6–8 Physics questions and 5–7 Mathematics questions.

Bear in mind that, as in Section 1, you are not allowed to use a calculator to answer this section. As such, you should always try to write your workings down. You won't get any marks for your workings, but under pressure even basic mathematical questions will become more difficult, so you can only benefit from using the spare pages provided.

Preparing for Section 2

Believe it or not, this section looks a lot worse than it actually is. The idea that the questions will be drawn from an enormous number of topics within Maths and the Sciences may seem horrifying, but in reality it's not too difficult to work out which areas to prepare. On the BMAT website, there is a list of subjects which the exam will *not* assess you on; these include:

• Green plants as organisms

• Useful products from organic sources

• Useful products from metal ores and rocks

• Useful products from air

• Changes to the Earth and atmosphere

• The Earth and beyond

• Seismic waves

Essentially, this leaves questions relating to Human Biology, and basic Maths, Physics and Chemistry. You can look at the GCSE curricula on each of the major examinations boards' websites:

• AQA: www.aqa.org.uk

• Edexcel: www.edexcel.org.uk

• OCR: www.ocr.org.uk

They will give you a good idea of the range of questions you could be asked. Have a look through some GCSE past papers, which are available for download from the exam boards' websites or you may still have some of these lying around. Or brush up on your knowledge using GCSE textbooks. Whichever way you choose to revise, it's important to refresh your knowledge.

Practice papers of the BMAT are also available to download from the BMAT website directly. Visit www.BMAT.org.uk to ensure you are as fully prepared as possible.

Just like the rest of the BMAT, this section isn't designed to catch you out. You won't be asked anything that you couldn't possibly already know, and since you'll most likely be studying a range of Sciences at A-level anyway, you will probably have revisited many of the potential topics already. Remind yourself of some of the more common formulas and principles and you should be able to cover most of the relevant knowledge to succeed in this section.

Section 2: Worked examples

Example question 1: Biology

Study the following statements about viruses. Which statements are true?

1   They have a protein coat
2   They can cause cancer
3   They can cause TB
4   Their DNA can integrate into human DNA
5   They exist naturally in the body

A   1, 2 and 4
B   1, 2, and 5
C   1, 3, and 5
D   1 alone
E   1 and 2

Answer

Option 1   True, a virus has a protein coat. It is referred to as a capsid

Option 2   True, cervical cancer has been linked to Human Papilloma Virus. Girls are currently being vaccinated against this

Option 3   False, TB is a caused by a bacterial infection

Option 4   True, a common example is the Herpes Simplex Virus (cold sores), where the virus can lie latent in its host DNA, meaning you can never be cured

Option 5   False, it is bacteria that exist naturally in the body, such as the bacteria in our gut involved in the digestion of food.

The correct answer is A, as statements 1, 2 and 4 are true.

Example question 2: Maths

A frustrum of a cone is formed by cutting the top off a cone. The original cone has a base radius of 6cm and height of 10cm. The part of the cone removed has a base radius of 3cm and height of 5cm. What is the volume of the frustrum? Give your answer to the nearest cm³.

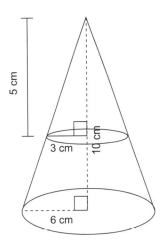

Answer

First we calculate the volume of the whole cone:

We take π to be 3 (as you are not allowed calculators)

Volume $= \frac{1}{3} \pi r^2 h$
$= \frac{1}{3} \times 3 \times 6^2 \times 10$
$= 360 \text{ cm}^3$

Then we calculate the volume of the small cone:

Volume $= \frac{1}{3} \pi r^2 h$
$= \frac{1}{3} \times 3 \times 3^2 \times 5$
$= 45 \text{ cm}^3$

We then subtract the volume of the small cone from that of the original cone to find the volume of the frustrum:

= 360 cm^3 − 45 cm^3
= 315 cm^3

Example question 3: Physics

A car with a weight of 8000N, travels 1,200 metres in a minute. Use the following equation to calculate the kinetic energy of the car. (Take the gravitational field strength as 10 N/kg).

Kinetic energy (J) = ½ mass (kg) × speed^2 (m/s)

A   320,000J
B   80,000J
C   160,000J
D   160,000kJ
E   320,000kJ

Answer

We first need to calculate the mass of the car:

Mass = weight in Newtons ÷ gravitational field strength (N/kg)
       = 8,000 ÷ 10
       = 800kg

We then need to calculate the speed of the car in m/s
Speed = distance (m) ÷ time (s)
       = 1200 ÷ 60
       = 20 m/s

So Kinetic energy of the car   = ½ 800 × 20^2
                                = 400 × 400
                                = 160,000J

The correct answer is C.

Example question 4: Chemistry

In which of the following reactions is copper reduced?

A $\quad$ $Fe + Cu^{2+} \longrightarrow Fe^{2+} + Cu$

B $\quad$ $2Cu + O_2 \longrightarrow 2CuO_2$

C $\quad$ $2CuO + C \longrightarrow 2Cu + CO_2$

D $\quad$ $CuO + H_2 \longrightarrow Cu + H_2O$

E $\quad$ $Cu + 2Ag^+ \longrightarrow Cu^{2+} + 2Ag$

Answer

When faced with an Oxidation/Reduction question remember the acronym OILRIG: Oxidation Is Loss of electrons, Reduction Is Gain of electrons.

Reduction is where an element gains electrons. In A, copper gains 2 electrons as it goes from Cu^{2+} to Cu ($Cu^{2+} + 2e^- \longrightarrow$ Cu), so A is a reduction.

A reduction reaction can also be defined as losing oxygen, as in C and D. The copper in CuO, is Cu^{2+} and upon reaction with carbon or hydrogen is reduced to Cu. So C and D are also reduction reactions of copper.

In B and E, copper is oxidised, as copper has lost two electrons ($Cu \longrightarrow Cu^{2+} + 2e^-$)

So the correct answers are A, C and D.

Chapter 5 Section 3: Writing Task

Overview of Section 3

During your time at university, you will come across many new or complex concepts and ideas. You may agree with some of them, and you may disagree with others, but the important point is how well you understand what you are reading and how well you can communicate your own views, opinions or ideas to your fellow peers. As a doctor or vet, this skill will be essential in both your day-to-day clinical work, as well as in activities such as teaching, research and presentations.

This section of the test requires you to write a short essay (limited to one side of A4) based on a statement or quote. You will have **30 minutes** in which to complete this section. You will be provided with three statements to choose from. Each will present an idea which you will have to assess, understand and critically argue, both for and against. The basic format for each statement will follow a similar pattern:

- Understanding – what do you understand the statement to mean?
- Argument – can you provide an argument to oppose the statement?
- Resolution – can you resolve the situation or give examples to demonstrate why the statement may or may not be true?

Unlike your A-level essays, you will not be required to demonstrate research or knowledge of specific facts or concepts. You will be presenting your own views, opinions and arguments based on what *you think* about the issues raised, so the emphasis is firmly on the way in which you approach the question. You should consider the following:

- Can you approach an argument from different perspectives?
- Can you clearly communicate your views and ideas?
- Can you resolve conflict between opposing arguments?
- Can you illustrate your argument with well-thought examples?

Once you have grasped these concepts, you should be in a much better position to attempt this section of the BMAT.

Preparing for Section 3

It may seem at first that this is a very difficult task to prepare for. It's true that you can't just learn to recite a whole load of facts and theories, but you can learn how to *approach* the questions in the right way. There are plenty of textbooks that cover how to think critically and formulate arguments; go to the library and read through a few to get an idea of the style and technique required for a good answer.

You should also be prepared to read around your studies; read journals, newspapers and medical websites to keep up-to-date with current clinical, legal or ethical issues in the world of medicine. Not only will this help with your current studies and give you something to include on your personal statement, you will hopefully acquire a good range of knowledge to draw on when answering the question. Make notes of your research, and *have an opinion!* You won't get great marks just for reciting verbatim the recent debate over stem cell research or repeating an article you read on human cloning. Understand how the issues you're reading about affect the real world, and come up with arguments as to why you do and don't agree with them. Even if you don't have the chance to use these specific examples within the exam, you'll at least get some practice in debating these kinds of issues and putting across your considered opinion in a clear and well-thought out way.

Finally, don't wait until a week before the exam to start frantically checking out journals or waking up at 7am every day to get the morning newspaper. Start your reading a couple of months before the exam and try to keep it going. Build up a good set of notes and resources and you'll have plenty to write about in the exam. The university may also ask you to elaborate on anything you discuss during the interview, so you'll definitely benefit from having an in-depth understanding of what you're writing about.

Tips for writing essays

Just as in Sections 1 and 2, you will be provided with a paper answer sheet in which to write your answer. The answer sheet is one side of A4; your answer can be no longer than the space provided, as no further answer sheets will be available. The length of your answer will obviously depend on the size of your handwriting, but you should be aiming to write around 300–350 words. You should also ensure that your writing is as neat as possible.

Plan ahead!

The fact that you have a limited space and time in which to compose your essay means that you will have to focus your ideas quickly and effectively. As with any other essay, the best way to do this is to plan ahead; there will be a blank sheet near the front of the exam paper where you can write notes – *use it*!

Get some key ideas written down and know what you're going to say so you don't have to start writing blindly. You'll have 30 minutes in total; since you're only writing 300–350 words, there shouldn't be a problem spending five to ten minutes ordering your thoughts coherently.

Choosing a question!

There won't be a 'right' or 'wrong' statement to choose; each statement will have its own complexities and pitfalls, so no one statement will be any more difficult than the other. Which statement you choose will be entirely up to you, so ensure you take a minute or two to read through the options and choose the statement you think you could fully answer in the best possible manner. The best approach to choosing a statement is to trust your gut instinct – if you look at a particular statement and immediately think 'I could write something about that', then it may be the best one to choose.

Read the question!

You've probably heard this a hundred times already regarding exams, but it's an important point to bear in mind. The BMAT isn't designed to trick you or catch you out. The questions are simple and to the point – all you need to do is make sure that you are answering the question that's in front of you. Each question will have a set of prompts, which are there to help you in setting your train of thought in the right direction. They will also provide you with a rough idea of how to structure your argument.

Get to the point!

In a normal essay you would be expected to refer to your research and explain, in detail, how you came to your conclusion. The BMAT essay is more focussed on reason and argument than presenting hard evidence. Since you won't have to worry about citing quotes or including insightful research, you can move quickly into addressing the question at hand. Bear in mind the following:

- Build your argument in a logical way; each sentence should follow into the next until you reach your conclusion
- Don't waste your word count – every sentence should be relevant to the question
- Have a conclusion! Don't let the essay just fade away into nothing right at the end. You don't have many words to play with, but your argument should certainly reach a satisfying conclusion.

Be coherent!

You've read the options, chosen a question and scribbled down an essay plan to get yourself started – a good start! All you need to do now is to transfer the words from your head, via your pen, to the answer paper. Sounds easy enough, but under pressure it's tempting to try and overdo it to squeeze a few more marks. Being able to write beautiful, flowing prose will certainly be an advantage, but you're not expected to write an essay of Shakespearian proportions. Too much flowery prose may obscure what was otherwise a perfectly good point. Avoid using complex terminology unless you're absolutely sure of what it means, and avoid unnecessarily long words – don't say 'hippopotomonstrosesquipedaliophobia' when what you mean is 'fear of long words'.

Check for errors

Where possible, you should leave a minute or two at the end of this section to go back and check through your essay for errors. When you're writing against the clock you're bound to make one or two spelling or grammatical errors, so it is worthwhile at the end to go back and check for any obvious mistakes. As discussed overleaf, you'll be marked on your clarity of language as well as content, so eliminating any grammatical errors can only work in your favour.

Section 3 Mark Scheme

When examining your answer, the assessors will mark your essay according to a set scale. The original scoring scale can be found at:

www.admissionstests.cambridgeassessment.org.uk/adt/ bmat/practice

We have included a summary of the scale below for quick reference.

Score	Description
0	The answer is completely irrelevant to the question asked or is missing
3	The answer does address the question in some way, and uses basically comprehensible English, but is incoherent, confused or does not address the question in the required manner
6	The answer addresses most parts of the question in a fairly logical way, but may be confused or use poor English; certain elements of the question may have been misunderstood, or the candidate may have provided a weak counter-argument

9	The answer addresses all elements of the question in a reasonably well-argued way and the counter-argument is rational and convincing, with good use made of material provided; the use of English is clear but may be slightly ineffective, and the argument may be slightly incoherent, with some elements potentially overlooked
12	The answer is good, with fewer weaknesses than answers with a score of 9
15	The answer is excellent; the argument is completely logical, clearly constructed and is written in complex and accurate English

Section 3 Worked Example

Let's have a look at an example question from Section 3:

1	**It is more important to know what sort of person has a disease than to know what sort of disease a person has** (Hippocrates) Write a unified essay in which you address the following: What do you think the author means by this statement? Can you suggest examples where it may be more important to understand the disease than the person? To what extent is it important to understand the personal qualities of your patients?

Okay, now let's break the question down and look at each part:

Write a unified essay

In a 'unified' essay, all of your arguments should support your essay. This may sound obvious, but it means that you need to define exactly what you are writing about beforehand, or your essay will quickly veer away from the central point.

What do you think the author means by this statement?

Note the key words – 'what do *you think*'. This is an easy way to start writing the essay. Just write about what you think it means – no tricks, no surprises, just write about your understanding of the statement.

Can you suggest examples where it may be more important to understand the disease than the person?

Simply agreeing with an idea or concept won't be enough to enable you to formulate a strong argument. You need to be able to look at a concept from all angles and present a counter-proposal, using different points of view to construct a well-rounded and considered argument.

To what extent is it important to understand the personal qualities of your patients?

Any essay needs a good conclusion to draw all of the points together. Now you've discussed what you think the statement means (and doesn't mean), you need to resolve your opposing arguments to explore what the statement is really addressing. This will be vital to presenting a logical and sensible conclusion.

Think about the statement presented and make some notes in the space below – how would you go about answering this question? Then see if your ideas match up to our example notes on the next page.

'It is more important to know what sort of person has a disease than to know what sort of disease a person has'

Notes:

Planning your answer

Let's start making some notes; the first step is to remind ourselves of the statement:

'It is more important to know what sort of person has a disease than to know what sort of disease a person has'

Now let's think about what this statement could mean. Don't forget that you will have a whole sheet of A4 in which to plan your answer, so use as much of the space as you need.

The simplest approach to planning your answer is to use the order of questions provided. Each sub-question within the main question provides a helpful 'anchor' for you to base your arguments on. You don't necessarily have to follow this approach rigidly, but under timed exam conditions it's a good idea to follow the most straightforward process to writing your answer.

There are a number of ways you could plan your answer. Some people may prefer to write a few sparse notes or keywords to link together the different aspects of their arguments. Others may prefer to draw diagrams to visualise their answers. Try out a few different techniques and see which way you find easiest.

For example, you could simply write notes or a basic flowchart in the order the question is asking you:

What does the statement mean?

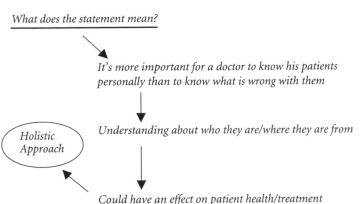

It's more important for a doctor to know his patients personally than to know what is wrong with them

Understanding about who they are/where they are from

Holistic Approach

Could have an effect on patient health/treatment

When is it more important to understand the illness?

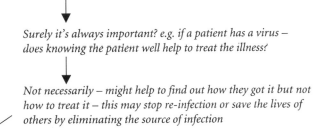

Surely it's always important? e.g. if a patient has a virus – does knowing the patient well help to treat the illness?

Not necessarily – might help to find out how they got it but not how to treat it – this may stop re-infection or save the lives of others by eliminating the source of infection

Practical knowledge important!

To what extent is it important to understand the personal qualities of your patients?

It is important but not necessarily more important than understanding the illness – without a good practical/medical understanding, the doctor cannot provide the necessary medical care

Need to use practical and personal skills together for best effect

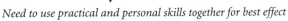

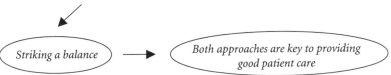

Striking a balance ⟶ *Both approaches are key to providing good patient care*

Whichever method you prefer, make sure you do make time to plan your answer out – don't get halfway through a question and realise you don't have anything to say!

Example answer

Now you've thought about the question and made a few notes, let's examine a possible answer:

The statement by Hippocrates describes something that, in modern medicine, would be called a 'holistic approach'. He is stating that simply understanding what is wrong with a patient is not sufficient to treat them; understanding a patient's personal situation is just as important to reaching a diagnosis: do they have allergies to medication? Do their living conditions or lifestyle have an effect on the illness? Managing a chronic illness, such as diabetes, is much easier if the doctor understands the patient's diet, alcohol intake, level of exercise, etc. Considering all of these points will help the doctor to reach a more accurate diagnosis.

However, it is important to remember that every doctor must possess relevant and up to date medical knowledge. Understanding a patient's situation is irrelevant if a doctor is unable to make the correct diagnosis and design an appropriate treatment plan. For example, while it is important to know how or where a patient contracted a virus, it is equally important that the doctor is able to identify the virus, prescribe the correct treatment and advise the patient on how to recover. Practical knowledge and skills are vital, and every doctor should work hard to ensure that his or her own knowledge is sufficiently up to date at all times.

> *A doctor needs to be able to understand both the patient and the disease they are treating and combine this knowledge to form a treatment plan for that particular patient. Possessing a good general medical knowledge is important, but without understanding the patient the doctor may suggest an inappropriate or ineffective course of action. Similarly, for a doctor to know about a patient's job or family life but not understand how to cure them of their illness would be a dangerous situation. It is not more important for a doctor to understand the patient, but it is an extremely important part of the treatment process.*

Note that we have used the prompts from the plan to structure our answer; each paragraph corresponds to one of the smaller questions asked as part of the original question, which has helped us to structure our answer with a solid 'beginning-middle-end' format. Let's look at each paragraph in turn and examine how we came to this answer.

Paragraph 1

> *The statement by Hippocrates describes something that, in modern medicine, would be called a 'holistic approach'. He is stating that simply understanding what is wrong with a patient is not sufficient to treat them; understanding a patient's personal situation is just as important to reaching a diagnosis: do they have allergies to medication? Do their living conditions or lifestyle have an effect on the illness? Managing a chronic illness, such as diabetes, is much easier if the doctor understands the patient's diet, alcohol intake, level of exercise, etc. Considering all of these points will help the doctor to reach a more accurate diagnosis.*

What do you think the author means by this statement?

In this opening statement we have detailed what we thought the statement meant, which is exactly what we were asked to do. To illustrate our understanding, we have included examples of where the statement may apply, for example, in understanding the lifestyle of a diabetes patient. This way, instead of simply stating the facts, we are constructing a suitable response based on how we understand the statement. Consider the following:

The statement by Hippocrates means that it is more important to understand the patient than to understand what is wrong with them.

This may answer the question in a very basic way – the student said what you think it means – but there's no real substance to the answer. They haven't displayed a good level of understanding or of being able to explore the concept instead of simply reciting what it means. Tie the statement in to something relevant, i.e. a real-life, applicable situation, in order to show that what you are saying isn't just something you've made up on the spot.

One thing to remember is not to force too much into your opening paragraph. Remember what you're working towards – a well-paced, flowing and balanced essay. Tackle each sub-question one at a time and make sure that each paragraph flows into the next until you reach your conclusion.

Paragraph 2

> *However, understanding a patient's situation is irrelevant if a doctor is unable to make the correct diagnosis and design an appropriate treatment plan. For example, while it is important to know how or where a patient contracted a virus, it is equally important that the doctor is able to identify the virus and prescribe the correct treatment. Similarly, for a surgeon operating to remove a complex tumour, anatomical knowledge and practical skills would take precedence over a personal connection with the patient. Practical knowledge and skills are vital, and every doctor should work hard to ensure that his or her own knowledge is sufficiently up to date at all times.*

Can you suggest examples where it may be more important to understand the disease than the person?

Here we've presented our counter-argument to the statement, which makes up the central part of our essay. Our argument is that, although we do not disagree with the original statement, practical skills and knowledge are also vital in diagnosing patients. In this way, we're not simply saying 'the original statement is wrong'; we're showing that we can build a good argument that takes all sides into account, which in turn helps us to work towards our conclusion in the final paragraph.

Bear in mind that the question specifically asks for you to *suggest examples* to support your argument. If you don't use an example of some kind, you will certainly sacrifice marks and lower your overall score for this section. This is why researching a wide variety of topics as part of your exam preparation is a good idea. Having a few 'real-life' case studies to call upon will give you some flexibility; you could use one example, or more if necessary. Be as specific as you can, but remember to keep your examples relevant – don't just wedge something in because you remember it, as you're being scored on the coherence of your argument.

Some people will find it easier than others to come up with examples. Not everyone is able to quote Einstein or Newton on demand, so work within what you know. If all else fails, keep it simple; a good quality answer with a simple example will score much better than an answer quoting word-perfect lines from Darwin's *Origin of Species*, but which makes absolutely no sense and is irrelevant to the question.

Paragraph 3

> *A doctor needs to be able to understand both the patient and the disease they are treating and combine this knowledge to form a treatment plan for that particular patient. Possessing a good general medical knowledge is important, but without understanding the patient the doctor may suggest an inappropriate or ineffective course of action. Similarly, for a doctor to know about a patient's job or family life but not understand how to cure them of their illness would be a dangerous situation. It is not more important for a doctor to understand the patient, but it is an extremely important part of the treatment process.*

To what extent is it important to understand the personal qualities of your patients?

Our final paragraph is where we have resolved the two counter-arguments presented in the first two paragraphs. We have presented a balanced and logical argument by reasoning that *both* sides of the argument are equally valid and must both be taken into account when diagnosing a patient. The conclusion is a logical progression from the previous paragraphs and neatly ties together the issues already raised (remember – a *unified* essay).

Pay close attention to the wording of this question, particularly '*To what extent*'. This could equally be worded as '*How far should*', or '*When is it*' or '*Why is it*'. The question is directing you to qualify your ideas rather than just stating a simple opinion. This is your invitation to take the points put forward in the first two paragraphs and to close the argument one way or another.

It may be, however, that you tend to agree with one point more than the other, or that you think all of the arguments are flawed – that's fine. You can argue in either direction, since there are no right or wrong answers to these questions, as long as you justify your point of view. The important thing is that, no matter what you believe, you are able to put across your views in a reasonable, convincing manner. For example:

A doctor should always focus on treating the physical symptoms of illness and should place less emphasis on understanding the patient. Successfully treating the illness is far more important than getting to know the patient or understanding their situation, and a doctor should not waste valuable time when they should be concentrating on treating patients.

Are you convinced? The writer has stated a lot of opinions but hasn't gone as far as to even try to justify them. The answer might get a couple of marks for being written in coherent English, but the argument itself is non-existent.

Section 3: Practice Questions

Now we've looked at Section 3 in detail, take a look at these example questions and apply the same reasoning to each to see if you can come up with an answer. You may find it useful to time yourself. You'll find our own notes on the following pages – see how yours compare.

1   **Intuition does not in itself amount to knowledge, yet cannot be disregarded by philosophers and psychologists** (Corliss Lamont)

What do you understand this statement to mean within a medical context?

Give examples to illustrate when intuition may be a beneficial influence on patient care and when it may be detrimental

How much emphasis should a clinician place on using their initiative when treating a patient?

2   **Medicine is driven by the sciences; the more we understand about science, the better medicine will become**

What is your understanding of this statement?

In what instances may the field of medicine not be directly affected by scientific developments and when is it reliant on such developments?

How far does progress within medicine depend on progress in the sciences?

3   **The doctor of the future will give no medicine but will interest his patients in the care of the human frame, in diet and in the cause and prevention of disease** (Thomas Edison)

What does this statement mean to you?

Using examples, discuss where it is important for a doctor to teach patients to look after themselves, and where it may be more important to treat the patient directly

To what extent is it important for doctors to promote good health through patient education?

Section 3: Example Answer 1

Intuition does not in itself amount to knowledge, yet cannot be disregarded by philosophers and psychologists
(Corliss Lamont)

What do you understand this statement to mean within a medical context?

- Intuition and knowledge are separate concepts but are not completely independent from one another
- Intuition is not knowledge in that it does not necessarily depend on proven or recognised factual information
- Even though intuition cannot replace medical knowledge and training, it cannot be disregarded in terms of patient care
- Intuition is what enables doctors to question situations and further the field of medicine

Give examples to illustrate when intuition may be a beneficial influence on patient care and when it may be detrimental

- Emergency or trauma situations – for example, a patient may present with unidentified bleeding after a car accident; in order to save their life, a surgeon may have to act without ordering the standard tests (X-rays, MRIs) and perform surgery without being fully prepared

- Using intuition
- Detrimental – doctor may be isolated and afraid to ask for help

How much emphasis should a clinician place on using their intuition when treating a patient?

- Dependent on situation i.e. A&E versus long term treatment plan
- Where possible facts should be established in order to make a decision, however
- The patient's care should be priority above all, and sometimes doctors do not have the luxury of time
- Where possible intuition should be used to debate decisions with colleagues to ensure correct decisions are made

Section 3: Example Answer 2

Medicine is driven by the sciences; the more we understand about science, the better medicine will become

What is your understanding of this statement?

- Medicine and science are inextricably linked; medicine depends on progress in the sciences and cannot progress of its own accord
- The statement could suggest that the roles of doctors and scientists are separate; that scientists work in one discipline, whilst doctors work in the other
- Alternatively, it could also suggest that doctors must incorporate the philosophy of a close relationship with science in order to further their own profession

In what instances may the field of medicine not be directly affected by scientific developments, and when is it reliant on such developments?

- Could depend on a definition of 'the sciences'; psychology and psychiatry could be influenced by the biological sciences (for example in linking psychopathic behavioural disorders to neurological conditions), and could also be associated with social sciences
- Most medical equipment is reliant on developments in science (e.g. MRIs, X-rays)
- Most advances in treatment are due to research by scientists (e.g. cancer treatment, heart disease and stem cell therapy); it could be argued medicine is reliant or directly affected by these.
- In order to treat a disease, it must be understood – e.g. in the treatment of Alzheimer's, until the pathway that leads to the build-up of protein deposits in the brain is understood how can doctors go about treating it? In this case medicine is reliant on scientific development.
- Third World countries have no access to the latest treatment advances

How far does progress within medicine depend on progress in the sciences?

- As a profession, medicine is something of a hybrid; it incorporates elements of the science, but also depends on other disciplines
- 'Clinical science' is closely related to medicine and draws upon many aspects of the 'classical' sciences.
- Evidence-based medicine relies on the discovery of both scientists and doctors to enable the development of new treatments or the refinement of existing approaches.

Section 3: Example Answer 3

The doctor of the future will give no medicine but will interest his patients in the care of the human frame, in diet and in the cause and prevention of disease
(Thomas Edison)

What does this statement mean to you?

- Progress in medicine places the emphasis firmly on the patient, not necessarily on the doctor
- The doctor does still carry responsibility, but in an educational context rather than through treatment and intervention
- Medicine and healthcare will eventually be the responsibility of the patient, and that patients will only resort to doctors in serious or unpreventable circumstances
- Prevention is better than a cure

Using examples, discuss where it is important for a doctor to teach patients to look after themselves, and where it may be more important to treat the patient directly

- Current debates about obesity suggest that it is important for any patient to take personal responsibility for their own actions; in most cases, obesity is related to a poor diet and lack of exercise
- Poor diet ultimately results in further medical complexities, such as diabetes (and all its related problems), high blood pressure and heart conditions; thus, an obese patient whose weight is their own responsibility could tie up resources and thus prevent others from receiving timely and costly treatment
- On the other hand, certain conditions (eating disorders and metabolic illnesses) could lead to patients becoming obese

through no fault of their own; regardless of diet, these patients require medical intervention or risk further illness or death

To what extent is it important for doctors to promote good health through patient education?

- Educating patients can only prove to be a benefit in the long run as it would take the strain off the medical infrastructure and enable doctors to treat those patients who are unable to simply help themselves
- However, doctors can never be completely removed from the equation; regardless of whether an illness is due to lifestyle or circumstance, doctors are duty bound to provide care wherever possible
- Ultimately, doctors will always be required to provide interventional treatment, regardless of how capable patients are of looking after their own health

Chapter 6 Full BMAT Mock

We would recommend that the best way to prepare for the BMAT is to complete a full practice paper, under timed conditions, in order to fully appreciate the nature of the exam you will be taking.

We recommend that you use spare sheets of A4 paper for your working out; in the real exam you will be able to use the blank sheets indicated as part of the test paper.

Remember that you are not permitted to use calculators during Sections 1 or 2, and that your answer for Section 3 should be no longer than one side of A4 paper. You should allow yourself no longer than two hours, as per the real exam, to gain the greatest benefit from this exercise. Remember the time allocations are as follows:

Section 1: Aptitude and Skills, 35 questions, 60 minutes

Section 2: Scientific Knowledge and Applications, 27 questions, 30 minutes

Section 3: Writing test, 1 essay question, 30 minutes

To make the most of this practice paper you can download a sheet to record your answers by visiting the Developmedica website (www.developmedica.com) and accessing the BMAT book product page.

Mock Section 1: Aptitude and Skills – 60 minutes

Question 1

To win a gold at the Olympic games in Judo, Satoshi Ishii from Japan had to beat six other players. How many people competed at the Olympic games in Judo?

A   60
B   32
C   64
D   128
E   124

Question 2

A virus-laden cream, to prevent the spread of MRSA, could be made available within the next two years. Scientists are at a highly advanced stage of developing the cream, which contains a combination of various viruses which target the MRSA bug. The cream is to be applied inside the noses of hospital patients. Once in the nose the viruses will fasten themselves onto the MRSA bacteria, and infuse the MRSA bacteria with their own genetic material. It has been proposed that viruses reproduce themselves, which suggests that repeated treatments may not be necessary, when compared to other treatments. The virus cream seems to be one of the latest ongoing examples of a resurgence of interest in bacteriophage viruses. It has been proposed that this specific form of treatment, involving the use of bacteriophages, may be a potential solution to the increasing problem of bacterial resistance to antibiotics.

What is inferred by the above passage?

A   A major advantage of the cream described is that it will only need to be applied twice, saving time and money

B   A specific treatment using the cream could prove a major advancement in the battle against antibiotic resistant bacteria

C   The cream will have uses in treatments against viral infections

D   The cream is in the early stages of development

E   The bacteriophage technology used is a form of bacteria

Question 3

The graph below shows the numbers of applicants to university over the past couple of years:

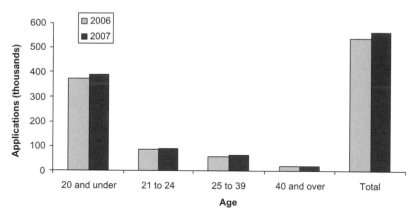

Which of the following statements can be deduced from the information given above:

1 Younger people are more likely to apply to university
2 More people are applying to university each year
3 More females apply than males

A   1 alone
B   1 and 2
C   2 and 3
D   All of the above
E   None of the above

Question 4

A clock comprising of six separately rotating number or letter panels shows the following time. What will be the total number of panel changes made to reach the time 01.22pm?

0	9:	2	2		
				A	M

A   248 rotations
B   271 rotations
C   171 rotations
D   280 rotations
E   210 rotations

Question 5

In 2003, losses in production due to mortality and morbidity associated with Coronary Heart Disease cost industry over £3,100 million, with around 30% of this cost specifically due to death and 70% due to illness in those of working age, a 25% rise when compared to costs incurred in 2002. The cost of informal care for people with Coronary Heart Disease was approximately £1,250 million in 2003.

Which one of the following best describes what is inferred by the passage?

A   CHD is a condition that does not need to be addressed

B   CHD poses a serious and increasing threat to industry

C   To save costs industry does not need to do anything about CHD

D   The cost of informal care of CHD sufferers is insignificant

E   Reducing death rates in CHD sufferers will decrease efficiency in industry

Question 6

Two motorbikes have a race at a track. One rides a Ducatti which has a maximum speed of 200mph, and the other rides a Honda which has a maximum speed of 150mph. The track is 10 miles long. When will the Ducatti lap the Honda?

A   After 11 minutes
B   After 12 minutes
C   After 13 minutes
D   After 14 minutes
E   After 15 minutes

Question 7

Matt wants to buy his wife Nicola a necklace for her birthday. He asks a jeweller for some advice. He learns from the jeweller that:

Diamond is more precious than ruby which is more precious than sapphire. Emerald is less precious than ruby but more precious than pearl.

Therefore, pearl must be less precious than:

A   Diamond and ruby but not necessarily less precious than sapphire
B   Diamond and sapphire but not necessarily ruby
C   Sapphire, but not necessarily ruby or diamond
D   Ruby but not necessarily diamond or sapphire
E   Ruby, diamond and sapphire

Questions 8, 9, 10 and 11 refer to the following information

The graph below shows the incidence of the most common cancers in 2007 in the UK per 100,000 of the population.

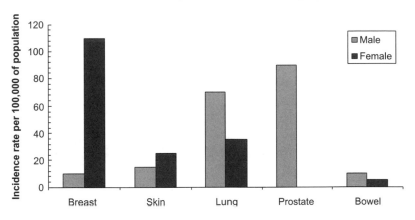

The population of the UK in 2007 was 60 million.

Question 8

How many people were diagnosed with breast cancer in 2007?

A   61,000
B   6,100
C   10,000
D   7,200
E   72,000

Question 9

What percentage of the male population was diagnosed with prostate cancer in 2007? (Assume that the population is equally distributed between males and females.)

A   0.09
B   0.9
C   0.045
D   0.45
E   9.5

YOU ARE NOW QUARTER OF THE WAY THROUGH THIS SECTION

Question 10

How many times more likely is a male to develop lung cancer than a female?

A   10
B   ½
C   3
D   2
E   20

Question 11

Which of the following pie charts is a correct representation of the incidence of cancer for both males and females per 100,000 people?

A

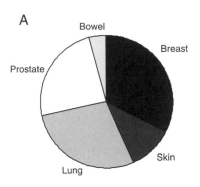

B

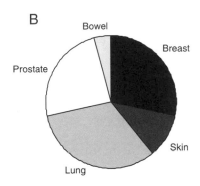

C

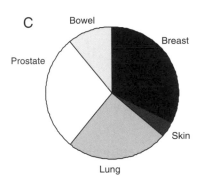

D

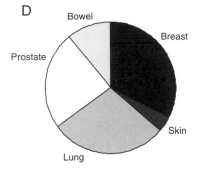

Question 12

Healthcare workers are at an increased risk of both fatal and non-fatal injuries, due to various factors ranging from violence within the workplace to apparatus being placed carelessly such as syringes and needles. Violence is increasing in severity and frequency in areas such as pharmacies, hospitals and community care facilities, and has now become a seemingly never-ending problem. It has been proposed that a complete resolution to such a problem would be to restrict the premature discharge of the chronically mentally ill from professional care services.

What is the main assumption in the above argument?

A   That needles do not pose a problem to healthcare staff

B   Discharging mentally ill patients earlier will protect healthcare workers from attack

C   That violence to healthcare staff is being caused by chronically mentally ill patients

D   Violence in hospitals is on the decrease

E   Syringes and needles are the same thing

Question 13

Which two of the following statements are equivalent:

A   James does not earn more than Peter
B   James earns at least as much as Peter
C   Peter earns at least as much as James
D   Peter earns more than James

Questions 14, 15, 16 and 17 refer to the passage below:

Read the following passage carefully

Although the underlying reasons are unclear, research conducted to date indicates an individual's degree of intelligence correlates with their degree of health and lifespan. It is thought that intelligence can influence the development of various approaches that can contribute to a better state of personal health and wellbeing, which include subscribing to the notion of following a vegetarian diet.

A cohort study recently published in the Journal of Healthy Eating by Dr Ed Smartz *et al* explores the degree to which intelligence influences an individual's development of initiatives to promote their own healthy lifestyle. In this study comprising 11,000 French males and females, it was shown that there was a positive correlation between childhood intelligence and going on to follow a subsequent vegetarian diet later in life. This relationship was shown to be independent of other potential influencing factors such as social class or academic achievement.

A retrospective analysis of five separate studies conducted has shown significantly (results normalised for smoking, age and sex) that individuals who follow a vegetarian diet are 69 per cent less likely to die than those that follow a non-vegetarian diet. A separate double blind study identified that higher ingestion of foods such as vegetables, wholemeal-based foods and certain types of fruit were linked to a reduced total mortality as a result of heart disease and lower incidences of cancer in individuals over 30 years old.

So looking back to the original question asked by Smartz *et al*; Does diet influence childhood intelligence and subsequent health in adulthood? A strong relationship was found in the British 1958 birth cohort, where a healthy diet score (which was based on the ratio of fresh fruit versus fried food consumption at the age of 33), together with a high educational achievement, significantly accounted for the association between childhood intelligence and becoming a vegetarian between the ages of 18–40 years. Therefore, if diet does have an effect on intelligence, which subsequently results in following what can be considered a more healthy, vegetarian lifestyle, this should surely lead to a decrease in health complications such as cancer and diabetes.

Intervention by public health authorities to encourage the following of consistently healthy lifestyles may have positive repercussions. Such an initiative could begin with parents being urged to encourage their children to eat more healthily, with the ultimate aim of them translating their healthy eating habits into adulthood. At the same time adults could be encouraged through positive education to realise the benefits of healthy eating and how these habits can be formed during childhood.

Question 14

Which of the below options best summarises what the above article infers?

A   Encouraging children to lead a healthy lifestyle will mean they live longer and are less likely to suffer from brain disease

B   The more intelligent an individual the less likely they will follow a vegetarian diet in later life

C   The more intelligent an individual in childhood the more likely they are to follow a vegetarian diet resulting in reduced risk of heart disease and cancer

D   Public health authorities have no obligation to intervene in the health of children and therefore are powerless to improve their quality of life

Question 15

What is the main assumption made in the article above?

A   Public health authorities are powerless to make a difference to the quality of life in adolescents through encouraging healthy lifestyles

B   Healthy eating and intelligence do not mean an individual will follow a vegetarian lifestyle

C   By being vegetarian individuals are more likely to be affected by heart disease and cancer

D   The more intelligent an individual is the more likely they are to follow a healthy lifestyle later in life

Question 16

According to the passage, in what year were the individuals in the British 1958 cohort assessed for healthy diet scores?

A   1994

B   1991

C   1958

D   1992

Question 17

Which of the following is the only true statement based on the information given in the passage?

A   11,000 French males were analysed as part of the cohort study

B   Results of the retrospective analysis of five studies were normalised for smoking, age and sex

C   One of the studies described was published in the Journal of Eating Healthily

D   69% of individuals are more likely to die if they follow a vegetarian diet

Question 18

There are 10 players in a netball team. The oldest is 16 years old, and the youngest 13 years old. There are twice as many 15 year olds as there are 14 year olds, and three times as many 16 year olds as 13 year olds. The median and modal age is 15. What is the mean age of the team?

A   15.0
B   15.1
C   14.9
D   13.9
E   14.1

YOU ARE NOW HALF WAY THROUGH THIS SECTION. YOU SHOULD IDEALLY HAVE 30 MINUTES REMAINING FOR THIS SECTION.

Question 19

The graph below shows the average cost of a barrel of crude oil ($) over the past seven years.

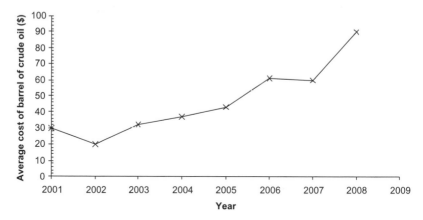

What was the average increase in price of crude oil between the years 2007 and 2008?

A   33%
B   50%
C   20%
D   25%
E   30%

Question 20

A bank has 100,000 customers, 60% of which have current accounts and 50% of which have credit cards. The bank sends a letter out to inform customers of rising interest rates. What is the maximum number of people who might receive two letters?

A   30,000
B   10,000
C   Can't tell
D   50,000
E   60,000

Question 21

The population of the United Kingdom is ageing. It has increased from 55.9 million in 1971 to 60.2 million in 2005. That is almost an 8% increase. However, this change is not spread out evenly across all age groups. In the last 30 or so years, the population aged 65 or over has increased from 13% to 16%. However, the percentage of the population under the age of 16 has declined from 25% in 1971 to 19% in 2005. Over the last 30 years, the mean age of the UK population has increased from 34.1 years in 1971 to 38.8 in 2005. This is principally due to reduced mortality in the older generation due to healthy living.

What can be inferred from the above?

A   The average age of the population is reducing due to mortality

B   The population dynamics have changed over a 50 year period

C   The percentage of elderly individuals in the population is increasing as they are living longer

D   The number of young people has decreased due to reduced fertility

Question 22

Eight friends go out for a meal.

They sit at a round table like the one below where the seating of certain individuals is illustrated.

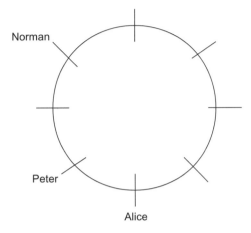

Katie is sitting to the right of Alice with Peter to her left.

Norman is to the left of Angela

Peter is sitting opposite Derek

Derek is sitting next to Katie and Janet

Angela is sitting next to Norman and Peter and opposite Katie

Which two people is June sitting next to?

A   Alice and Katie
B   Janet and Alice
C   Derek and Janet
D   Norman and Janet
E   Peter and Janet

Questions 23, 24, 25 and 26 refer to the data provided in the table below

The table below shows the salaries and monthly outgoings of the staff of a small company:

	Annual Salary (£)	Monthly outgoings (£)
James	42,000	2,200
Peter	25,000	1,900
Sarah	36,000	2,000
Louise	21,000	1,500
Frankie	25,000	1,400
John	30,000	1,800
Kevin	31,000	1,700

The annual salaries are given before income tax which is calculated at 20%.

Question 23

What is the average salary of the staff before tax?

A   £25,000
B   £33,000
C   £30,000
D   £27,000
E   £17,000

Question 24

Whose monthly outgoings are greater than their income after tax?

A   Louise and John
B   Peter and Louise
C   James and Louise
D   James and John
E   Peter and John

Question 25

The longer the staff have worked with the company the greater their pay. According to the graph below who is grossly over paid?

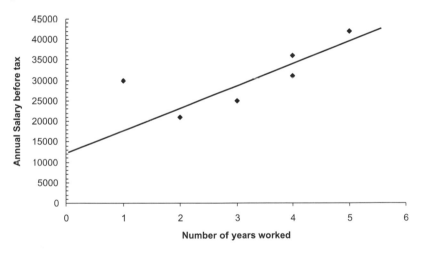

A   Kevin
B   James
C   Peter
D   John
E   Frankie

Question 26

Louise receives a 10% pay rise. After income tax has been deducted together with her monthly outgoings, how much can she expect to save each month?

A   £400

B   £600

C   £425

D   £154

E   £40

Question 27

Starting with the whole number in the furthest left column calculate the correct answer by following each instruction.

126	2/9 of this	× 3 ¼	6/13 of this	400% of this	5/12 of this	less 20%	62.5% of this	× 2 ¹/₇	−39

What is the final product?

YOU ARE NOW THREE QUARTERS OF THE WAY THROUGH THIS SECTION

Question 28

To qualify for Maternity Allowance an employee must be, or have recently been, either an employed or self-employed earner. The majority of people who qualify for leave will also qualify for pay, and vice versa. All employees who are parents to new babies have a right to statutory leave with pay. However, there are a few legal clauses. For instance, the privileges relating to time off for antenatal care, to maternity leave and to protection against detriment or unfair dismissal in connection with maternity leave do not apply to the following groups: members of the police force, MPs, the judiciary and certain types of company directors, or to masters or crew members engaged in share fishing paid solely by how much stock they have caught.

Which one of the following statements is true?

A   Firemen are excluded from privileges such as maternity leave and protection against unfair dismissal

B   You can only qualify for maternity leave if you have been employed

C   The rules relating to maternity leave do not apply to members of the police force

D   All fishermen are entitled to time off for antenatal care

E   All types of company directors are excluded from maternity leave

Question 29

A mobile phone company charges its customers a standard connection fee for each call made together with a standard rate per minute. A customer made two phone calls in a day, one for six minutes and was charged £2.65, and one for 15 minutes and was charged £5.80.

What is the connection fee and standard rate per minute?

Question 30

A local newsagent delivers papers to 60 houses. He delivers at least one item, but no more than three items to each house. 50% of the houses have a Sunday paper delivered, 60% a Saturday newspaper, and 30% a weekly magazine delivered.

Which two of the statements below must be true?

A   At least 6 people have both a Saturday and Sunday newspaper delivered.

B   At least 6 people do not have a Saturday or Sunday newspaper delivered

C   No more than 18 people have a magazine and Sunday newspaper delivered

Question 31

The Newcastle and Scottish Brewery has blamed the unpredict-able weather for their drop in profits for the year 2009. Statistics show last year's net profits of £76 million had dropped by 9% in the first six months of this year compared to the same period the previous year. The wet weather has been prominent throughout summer and, due to the fact that there is no large sporting event, such as the Rugby World Cup, to increase sales, this has led to a further 4.3% drop for the remainder of the year. The chairman of Newcastle Breweries has claimed that the continuation of this bad weather in the UK and France will make it most challenging to reach this year's target.

Which one of the following best describes the main conclusion of the passage?

A   The Newcastle and Scottish Brewery has made a loss of 19% compared to last year's net profits

B   The reason targets have been reached by Newcastle and Scottish Brewery is due in part to there being a Rugby World Cup

C   An upturn in the weather will ensure that Newcastle and Scottish Brewery hit their target

D   It is unlikely that Newcastle and Scottish Brewery will hit their targets this year

E   Bad weather in the US has caused a loss in revenue for the Newcastle and Scottish Brewery

Question 32

Milly rowed on an indoor rowing machine for one hour. In the first 20 minutes she rowed 6,000m. Her muscles then began to become tired and the distance she rowed in the next 20 minutes decreased by 5%. When she had 20 minutes left to go the adrenaline in her system kicked in and despite fatigue she managed to increase the distance travelled by 10% compared to that she rowed between 20 and 40 minutes.

How much further did Milly row in the final 20 minutes compared to the first 20 minutes?

A   4.2%
B   5.7%
C   2.7%
D   4.5%
E   2.9%

Question 33

The following graph shows the journey made by a lorry delivering goods to a supermarket.

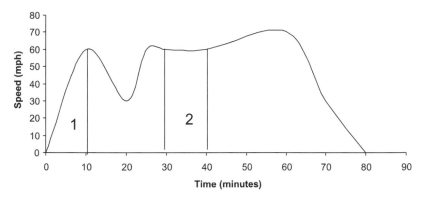

The area labelled 1 is half that labelled 2.

Which of the two following statements must be true:

A   The distance travelled between 0 and 10 minutes is half that travelled between 30 and 40 minutes

B   The lorry was travelling twice as quickly during 30–40 minutes as during 0–10 minutes

C   The average speed between 30 and 40 minutes is twice that of the average speed between 0 and 10 minutes

D   The lorry travelled quicker during the first 10 minutes than it did during 30–40 minutes of its journey

Question 34

A security guard has a code for the door to a store cupboard. He has many codes and struggles to remember them all. Instead of writing the codes down he writes clues to help him remember the codes.

1	2	3
4	5	6
7	8	9
	0	

The store cupboard code has 5 digits. He knows that:

No digit appears more than once in the code
The first digit is 2
The third digit is directly below the second
The fourth digit plus the first digit is the same as the third digit
The sum of the digits is 29

What is the final digit of the code?

A   7
B   8
C   5
D   0
E   3

Question 35

James uses SmartAbs gym seven days a week, visits ProBowl to go bowling on a Wednesday and Friday and swims at Riversmeet Leisure Centre on Sunday. Joe has a weekend only membership at SmartAbs gym where he only ever swims. During the week he goes to Riversmeet Leisure Centre for spinning classes on a Monday, Wednesday and Friday and goes bowling at ProBowl every Saturday night. John has a student membership at SmartAbs gym meaning he is restricted to using the gym Sunday to Thursday between the hours of 9am and 4pm, is a member of ProBowl which he visits every Saturday to play pool without fail and enjoys attending spinning classes on a Wednesday at Riversmeet Leisure Centre.

On one occasion all three individuals are present in a changing room at one of the above venues at the same time. Assuming that each individual above must use the changing facilities whenever they visit any of the above facilities, which one of the following is true

A   They are all attending spinning classes
B   It is a Sunday
C   They must be at the Riversmeet Leisure Centre
D   The time must be 9.30pm
E   It is a Saturday

Mock Section 2: Scientific Knowledge and Applications – 30 minutes

Question 1
The following are chemicals involved in digestion:

A   Carbohydrase
B   Bile
C   Protease
D   Lipase

From the above enter the chemical which:

(i)   Neutralises stomach acid
(ii)   Converts Proteins into Amino acids
(iii)   Is called Amylase
(iv)   Produces Fatty acids

Question 2
A packet of wine gums contains 3 red, 4 black and 5 green gums. Two gums are taken at random. What is the probability they will both be the same colour?

A   38/132
B   19/66
C   47/144
D   19/72
E   5/12

Question 3

Isotopes are defined as atoms which have the same number of protons but different numbers of neutrons.

$$^{12}_{6}\text{C}$$

Carbon 12 is the most common isotope of carbon. Considering the mass and atomic numbers, which of the options given below could also be an isotope of carbon?

	Mass	Atomic number
A	12	5
B	7	12
C	12	7
D	13	6
E	6	13

Question 4

A young girl places her hand in hot water. She immediately jumps back. Place the following series of events in the correct order, starting with the stimulus (heat) and finishing with the response (to move her hand).

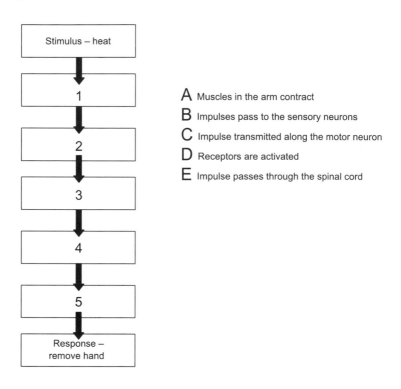

A Muscles in the arm contract

B Impulses pass to the sensory neurons

C Impulse transmitted along the motor neuron

D Receptors are activated

E Impulse passes through the spinal cord

Question 5

The volume of a cone is given by the formula:

$V = \frac{1}{3} \pi r^2 h$

Rearrange the formula to make r the subject.

Question 6

The kidneys are important organs responsible for maintaining the homeostatic balance of body fluids. How do the kidneys maintain blood pressure?

A By controlling the amount of ions such as sodium reabsorbed

B By releasing ADH

C By removing waste products from the body

D By regulating the amount of water reabsorbed into the blood

E By removing potassium from the blood

Question 7

A bullet is fired from a gun. An average force of 5000N acts for 0.01 seconds on a bullet with a mass of 50g.

The change in momentum can be calculated using the following equations:

Change in momentum = $mv - mu$

where m = mass of the bullet

   u = initial velocity of the bullet

   v = final velocity of the bullet

and

Force (N) = Change in momentum (kg m/s) ÷ Time (s)

At what speed is the bullet travelling when it is fired?

A 1000m/s

B 1m/s

C 2500m/s

D 250m/s

E 100m/s

Question 8

The diagram below shows a triangle *OAB*

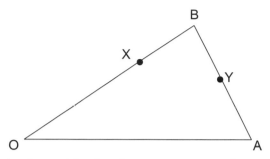

Y is the midpoint between AB, X lies on the line so that OX : OB = 2 : 1.

If $\overrightarrow{OA}$ = a, and $\overrightarrow{OB}$ = b, what in terms of a and b is the vector $\overrightarrow{XY}$.

A   5/6b − 1/2a

B   3/2a − 7/6b

C   −1/6b + 1/2a

D   4/6b − 1/2a

E   2/3b + a

Question 9

Use the table below to calculate the energy change of the reaction below.

$$CH_4 + 2O_2 \longrightarrow CO_2 + 2H_2O$$

Bond	Energy (kJ/mole)
C–C	350
C–H	400
O–H	450
O=O	500
C=O	800
C=C	600

A   800kJ
B   −800kJ
C   1,000kJ
D   −1,000kJ
E   500kJ

Question 10

Cystic fibrosis is a genetic disease which causes an excess of mucus to be produced in the lungs. It is caused by a faulty gene which is recessive. Study the family tree below. Which family members are definitely carriers of the faulty gene?

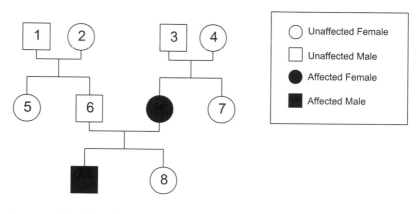

A   3 + 4 + 6 + 7

B   3 + 4 + 6

C   3 + 4 + 6 + 7 + 8

D   either 1 or 2 and either 3 or 4 + 6

E   either 1 or 2 and 3 + 4 + 6

Question 11

A square has a length $2\sqrt{5} + \sqrt{3}$ cm. What is the area of the square?

A $26 + 4\sqrt{10}$ cm^2
B $23 + 4\sqrt{15}$ cm^2
C $26 + 4\sqrt{25}$ cm^2
D $23 + 4\sqrt{25}$ cm^2
E $23 + 2\sqrt{15}$ cm^2

Question 12

A car has a mass of 700kg. It accelerates from 5m/s to 10m/s in 7 seconds. What is the driving force of the engine?

A   1400N
B   4900N
C   500N
D   100N
E   980N

Question 13

The diagram below shows a human heart.

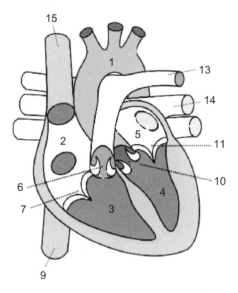

Which route is taken by oxygenated blood returning to the heart from the lungs?

A $14 \rightarrow 5 \rightarrow 11 \rightarrow 4 \rightarrow 10 \rightarrow 1$

B $13 \rightarrow 5 \rightarrow 11 \rightarrow 4 \rightarrow 10 \rightarrow 1$

C $15 \rightarrow 2 \rightarrow 7 \rightarrow 3 \rightarrow 6 \rightarrow 13$

D $15 \rightarrow 2 \rightarrow 3 \rightarrow 4 \rightarrow 5 \rightarrow 1$

E $1 \rightarrow 10 \rightarrow 4 \rightarrow 11 \rightarrow 5 \rightarrow 14$

Question 14

The diagram below shows a hydraulic breaking system. If a force of 5N is applied to the pedal, what force will be transferred on to the break pad?

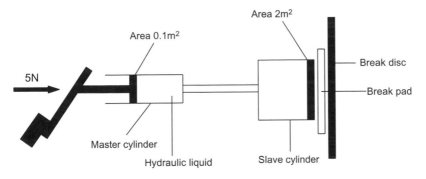

Question 15

Below are three wine glasses. All have a diameter of 8cm and the depth of B and C is 4cm. (Take π to equal 3.)

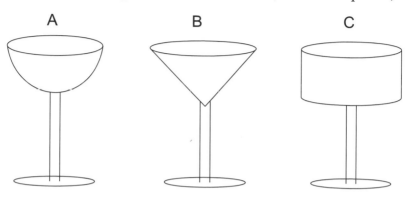

Which two of the following statements are true about the volumes of the glasses?

A   A>B >C
B   A>B but <C
C   B>A but <C
D   C>A but <B
E   A<C but >B

Question 16

The graph below shows a journey a cyclist made.

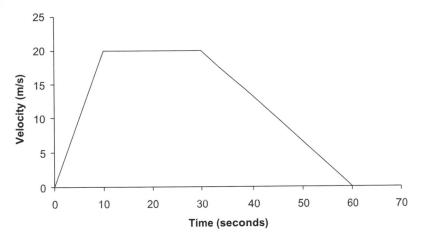

What distance was travelled by the cyclist?

A   100m

B   200m

C   1,300m

D   800m

E   1,200m

Question 17

Enzymes are biological catalysts which occur naturally in our bodies. Which of the following statements about enzymes are true:

A   They are sensitive to temperature and pH
B   They are used in the cheese making industry
C   The higher the temperature, the quicker they work
D   They increase the activation energy of a reaction
E   They are used in washing powder

Question 18

Calculate the mass in grams of iron produced when 40g of iron III oxide is reduced completely by aluminium. (M_r Fe = 56, O = 16, Al = 27)

$$Fe_2O_3 + 2Al \longrightarrow 2Fe + Al_2O_3$$

Question 19

The table below shows the effect of smoking and age on the death rate from Coronary Heart Disease (CHD).

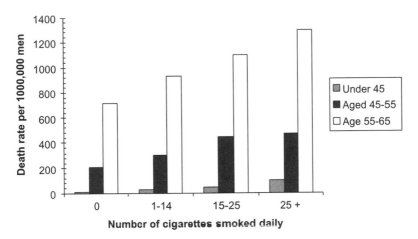

Why does smoking increase the risk of CHD? (Select the answers which are true.)

A   It raises blood cholesterol and blood pressure which can lead to arteriosclerosis

B   The nicotine the cigarettes contain stops the heart from working properly

C   Carbon monoxide released by the cigarettes reduces the amount of oxygen the red blood cells can transport to tissues

D   It prevents people exercising. This may lead to obesity which is a risk factor for CHD

E   Tar builds up in the arteries, reducing the flow of blood to the heart

Question 20

The graph below shows the decay of a radioactive substance.

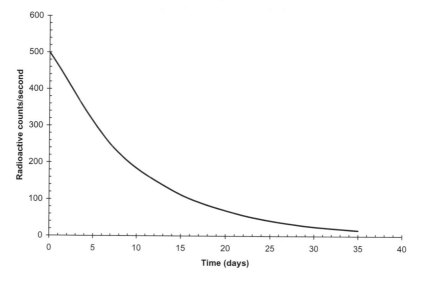

What is the half life of the substance?

A 35 days
B 5 days
C 7 days
D 10 days
E 9 days

Question 21

What values of a, b, c and d are required to balance the following equation?

$$aI_2 + bNa_2S_2O_3 \longrightarrow cNaI + dNa_2S_4O_6$$

Question 22

After eating a meal our blood sugar levels change. What happens in the body to control the blood sugar levels after eating?

	Blood sugar level	Hormone released	Effect of hormone
A	High	Insulin	Converts glucose into glycogen
B	High	Insulin	Converts glycogen into glucose
C	High	Glucagon	Converts glycogen into glucose
D	Low	Glucagon	Converts glycogen into glucose
E	Low	Insulin	Converts gulcose into glycogen

Question 23

A step down transformer has two coils. The voltage across the primary coil, which has 1000 turns, is 230V. Calculate the voltage across the secondary coil which has 100 turns.

Question 24

Molecular cloning is used in medicine to create identical copies of a DNA sequence. Which of the following is not an application or form of cloning?

A   Repopulation of endangered species
B   Creating genetically modified crops
C   Asexual reproduction
D   Generating new tissues and organs for transplants
E   IVF

Question 25

Solve the following equation

$$1 - \frac{(3x + 7)}{2} = \frac{(x + 4)}{4}$$

Question 26

The boxes labeled A-E below show the events involved in mitosis. List the events in the correct order beginning with E.

A Cytoplasm divides

B Chromatids separate

C Chromosomes align on the equator of the spindle

D Nuclear envelope disappears

E Chromosomes condense and become visible

Question 27

The graphs below show the resistance of certain electrical components. The dotted line in each graph represents a control using normal wire at constant temperature, and no other components. Here the current is directly proportional to the voltage.

Use the table on the next page to identify the components that give the solid lines in the graphs below.

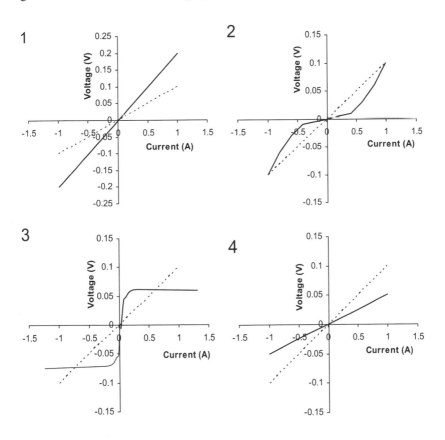

	1	*2*	*3*	*4*
A	Diode	Reduced Temperature	Filament bulb	Increased wire length
B	Increased wire length	Diode	Filament bulb	Increased Temperature
C	Decreased wire length	Filament bulb	Diode	Reduced Temperature
D	Increased Temperature	Filament bulb	Diode	Decreased wire length
E	Increased wire length	Diode	Filament bulb	Reduced Temperature

Mock Section 3: Writing Task- 30 minutes

ANSWER ONE OF THE QUESTIONS BELOW IN THE
SPACE PROVIDED ON THE ANSWER SHEET.

1   *'Body and soul cannot be separated for purposes of
    treatment, for they are one and indivisible. Sick minds
    must be healed as well as sick bodies'.*
    (C. Jeff Miller)

    What do you understand this statement to mean?

    Present examples to illustrate where conditions of mind
    and body are directly connected, and where they must
    be dealt with separately

    How would you propose the conflict between the
    treatment of physical and psychological illnesses be
    resolved?

2   *'A little knowledge that acts is worth infinitely more
    than much knowledge that is idle'.*
    (Kahlil Gibran)

    What do you think the above statement implies?

    Demonstrate through examples where acting on a small
    amount of knowledge may be less helpful than not
    acting on a wealth of knowledge

    To what extent should a clinician prioritise action over
    investigation?

3   *'A person cannot know more than they have experienced; without experience, a person cannot understand that which they know'*.

Explain in your own words what this statement suggests.

Give examples of how different levels of knowledge and experience, or lack thereof, could affect patient care

How far do you believe that knowledge and experience are dependent on one another?

Chapter 7 Full BMAT Mock Test Answers: Section 1

Question 1

Satoshi Ishii beat 6 players, therefore he must have played 6 rounds

There are two players in each round, so there must be

$2^6 = 2 \times 2 \times 2 \times 2 \times 2 \times 2$
$ = 64$ players

Therefore, the correct answer is C

Question 2

A. Incorrect

A major advantage of the cream described is that it will only need to be applied twice, saving time and money

The passage suggests that due to the nature of viruses replicating, the cream may only need to be applied once and that repeated treatments may not be necessary which contradicts the statement above. This option is therefore incorrect.

B. Correct

Using the cream could prove a major advancement in the battle against antibiotic resistant bacteria

The concluding sentence states that this form of treatment may be a potential solution to the increasing problem of antibiotic resistance in bacteria. This option therefore best describes what is inferred by the passage.

C. Incorrect

The cream will have uses in treatments against viral infections.

The passage clearly states that the cream is a form of bacterio-phage virus that can be used against bacterial infections not viral infections. This option is therefore incorrect.

D. Incorrect

The cream is in the early stages of development

The opening sentences state that the cream could be made available in the next two years and is at a highly advanced stage of development. This contradicts what this option states and is therefore incorrect.

E. Incorrect

The bacteriophage technology used is a form of bacteria.

As the passage states a bacteriophage is a form of virus and not bacteria this option is therefore incorrect.

The correct answer is B.

Question 3

Taking each point in turn:

1. **Younger people are more likely to apply to university:** As the difference between the number of younger people applying to university (20 and under), in 2006 and 2007 and older people (21 and above) is so significant. We can deduce that this statement is true.

2. **More people are applying to University each year:** As we are only given two years of data we cannot determine whether this is true, as in 2005 there could have been more applications than in 2006, and in 2008 there may be less than 2007. In order to determine this we need data from at least three years to establish a trend, so this statement cannot be proven.

3. **More females apply than males:** We are given no information about the split between male and female applications so cannot say whether this is true or not, so the statement cannot be proven.

The correct answer is A, only statement 1 can be proven.

Question 4

First panel rotates: $\times 2$
Second panel rotates: $\times 4$
Third panel rotates: 6×4
Fourth panel rotates: $10(4 \times 6)$
Fifth panel rotates: $\times 1$
Sixth panel rotates: $\times 0$
                      Total $= 271$ rotations

Therefore, the correct answer is Option B, 271

Question 5

A. Incorrect

CHD is a condition that does not need to be addressed

The theme of the passage revolves around the serious threat CHD poses to industry and certainly does not paint a picture of CHD being an issue that can be left alone. This option is therefore incorrect.

B. Correct

CHD poses a serious and increasing threat to industry

This option best describes what is inferred by the passage in terms of the effects of CHD on industry becoming increasingly worse. This option is therefore the best statement which describes what is inferred by the passage.

C. Incorrect

To save costs industry does not need to do anything about CHD

The passage states that CHD cost industry £3,100 million in 2003 and is an increase of 25% of the previous year. Therefore it would be incorrect to conclude that the passage implies that nothing needs to be done about CHD.

D. Incorrect

The cost of informal care of CHD sufferers is insignificant

£1,250 million is hardly an insignificant amount of money when describing the cost of informal care of sufferers of CHD and therefore this option is incorrect as it does not best describe what the article infers.

E. Incorrect

Reducing death rates in CHD sufferers will decrease efficiency in industry

This is not a plausible option because if death rates were reduced in CHD sufferers you would expect the efficiency to increase not decrease. This option is therefore incorrect.

Question 6

We need to calculate how long it takes each bike to complete a lap:

For the Ducatti:

Time = Distance ÷ Speed

   $= 10 \div 200$

   $= 1/20$ of an hour

   $= 3$ minutes per lap.

For the Honda:

Time = Distance ÷ Speed

   $= 10 \div 150$

   $= 1/15$ of an hour

   $= 4$ minutes per lap.

So the Ducatti will finish lap 1 after 3 minutes, lap 2 after 6 minutes, lap 3 after 9 minutes, **lap 4 after 12 minutes**, lap 5 after 15 minutes and so on.

The Honda will finish lap 1 after 4 minutes, lap 2 after 8 minutes, **lap 3 after 12 minutes**, and lap 4 after 16 minutes.

So after 12 minutes the Honda will be lapped by the Ducatti. Therefore the correct answer is B, after 12 minutes.

Question 7

Using the information we are given we can list the stones in order of preciousness:

Diamond
Ruby
Sapphire

We know that emerald is below ruby and is more precious than pearl, but we do not have any information about whether it is more or less precious than sapphire, therefore the correct answer is A.

Question 8

From the graph we can deduce that 110 females and 10 males, a total of 120 people in every 100,000 are diagnosed with breast cancer. We are told the population of the UK is 60 million. A simple scale up calculation is required.

So if 120 people in every 100,000 people are diagnosed

1,200 in every 1,000,000 are diagnosed

In a population of 60 million, there must be $1,200 \times 60 = 72,000$ people.

Therefore the correct answer is E.

Question 9

As prostate cancer only affects males, the population at risk is half of 60 million, 30 million. So to calculate what percentage of the male population was diagnosed with prostate cancer in 2007, we first need to calculate how many men were diagnosed.

We do this as we did for the previous question:

The graph shows there are 90 in every 100,000 people suffering with prostate cancer this equates to 900 in every million people.

So in a population of 30 million (males only) there are 900×30 = 27,000 males diagnosed.

To express this as a fraction of the population of males:

$(27,000 \div 30,000,000) \times 100$

$= (27 \div 30,000) \times 100$

$= (9 \div 10,000) \times 100$

$= 9 \div 100$

$= 0.09\%$ of the male population was diagnosed with prostate cancer in 2007.

Therefore the correct answer is A.

Question 10

We can deduce from the graph that 70 out of 100,000 men are diagnosed with lung cancer compared with 35 out of 100,000 females.

This means that twice as many men are diagnosed with lung cancer than females. They are therefore twice as likely to develop lung cancer than females. The correct answer is D.

Question 11

We need to look at the original graph and determine which cancers are more prominent:

For breast cancer 10 males + 110 females = 120 people per 100,000

For skin cancer 15 males + 45 females = 40 people per 100,000

For lung cancer 70 + 35 = 105 people per 100,000

For prostate = 90 people per 100,000

For bowel = 10 + 5 = 15 people per 100,000

So the sections of the pie chart starting from the largest to the smallest should be expressed in the following order:

Breast, lung, prostate, skin, bowel.

We simply look for the chart which expresses this correctly.

The correct answer is A.

Question 12

A. Incorrect

That needles do not pose a problem to healthcare staff

The passage clearly states that healthcare workers are being placed at an increased risk of both fatal and non-fatal injuries due to a range of factors including leaving needles carelessly. This option is therefore incorrect.

B. Incorrect

Discharging mentally ill patients earlier will protect healthcare workers from attack

The passage clearly states that it is the early release of mentally ill patients from professional care services that is resulting in increased violence to healthcare workers in various healthcare settings. This option is therefore incorrect.

C. Correct

That violence to healthcare staff is being caused by chronically mentally ill patients

The main assumption of the passage is that the violence to healthcare workers is being caused by chronically mentally ill patients who are being released early and that delaying their release will reduce the high incidence of violence. This is therefore the correct answer.

D. Incorrect

Violence in hospitals is on the decrease

The passage states that violence towards healthcare professionals is increasing in severity and frequency. This option is therefore incorrect.

E. Incorrect

Syringes and needles are the same thing

The focus of the passage is not whether syringes and needles are the same thing so this is irrelevant to the argument relating to violence. This is therefore an incorrect option.

Question 13

A.   James does not earn more than Peter, so he could earn the same as, or less than Peter. We can write this as James ≤ Peter

B.   James earns at least as much as Peter, so he could earn the same as, or more than Peter. We can write this as James ≥ Peter

C.   Peter earns at least as much as James, so he could earn the same as, or more than James. We can write this as Peter ≥ James

D.   Peter earns more than James. We can write this as Peter > James

So we have the following inequalities:

A.   James ≤ Peter
B.   James ≥ Peter
C.   Peter ≥ James
D.   Peter > James

We can restate the statement C by putting James first.

James ≤ Peter

which is equivalent to A

therefore A and C are equivalent

Question 14

Which of the below statements best summarises what the above article infers?

Option A. Incorrect

Encouraging children to lead a healthy lifestyle will mean they live longer and are less likely to suffer from brain disease

Although encouraging children to follow a healthy lifestyle may well result in them living longer the passage does not infer this and certainly does not mention any form of brain disease.

Option B. Incorrect

The more intelligent an individual the less likely they will follow a vegetarian diet in later life

In the second paragraph it is stated that there is a positive correlation between childhood intelligence and following a vegetarian diet, inferring that children are more likely to follow a diet of this type.

Option C. Correct

The more intelligent an individual in childhood the more likely they are to follow a vegetarian diet resulting in reduced risk of heart disease and cancer

In the second paragraph it is clearly stated that there is a positive relationship between childhood intelligence and following a vegetarian lifestyle. In the third paragraph a double blind study is described. When certain types of wholemeal foods, fruits and vegetables are ingested by individuals lower incidences of cancer and heart disease are observed. This option therefore best summarises what the passage infers.

Option D. Incorrect

Public health authorities have no obligation to intervene in the health of children and therefore are powerless to improve their quality of life

In the final paragraph it states that intervention by the public health authorities may have positive repercussions through a number of initiatives which contradicts the above statement, making it incorrect.

Question 15

Which statement best describes the main assumption made in the article above?

Option A. Incorrect

Public health authorities are powerless to make a difference to the quality of life in adolescents through encouraging healthy lifestyles

The final paragraph clearly describes initiatives the health authorities could implement to promote healthy lifestyles in children through the education of parents to urge their children to eat more healthily. This option is therefore incorrect.

Option B. Incorrect.

Healthy eating and intelligence do not mean an individual will follow a vegetarian lifestyle

Paragraph four states that the higher an individual's healthy eating score, which reflects the degree to which an individual follows a healthy diet, the more likely they are to follow a vegetarian lifestyle and be healthier, therefore contradicting the above option.

Option C. Incorrect

By being vegetarian individuals are more likely to be affected by heart disease and cancer

In paragraph three individuals who follow a diet high in wholemeal and fruit content are less likely to develop heart disease or cancer which suggests this option is incorrect.

D. Correct

The more intelligent an individual is the more likely they are to follow a healthy lifestyle later in life

This is really the main thrust of the passage which relies on the hypothesis stated in the opening paragraph that increased childhood intelligence leads to a healthy lifestyle later in life.

Question 16

According to the passage, in what year were the individuals in the British 1958 cohort assessed for healthy diet scores?

The correct answer is Option B as 1991 is the year that the individuals would have been in their 33rd year.

Questions 17

Which of the following is the only true statement based on the information given in the passage?

A. Incorrect

11,000 French males were analysed as part of the cohort study

In the second paragraph it clearly states that 11,000 males and females were included in the cohort study. Therefore this statement cannot be true because there must have been at least one female present in the cohort meaning that at the greatest there could only be 10,999 males present. This option is therefore incorrect.

B. Correct

Results of the retrospective analysis of five studies were normalised for smoking, age and sex

In the third paragraph, which describes a retrospective analysis, it clearly states in brackets that the results were normalised for smoking, age and sex. This is therefore the correct answer.

C. Incorrect

One of the studies described was published in the Journal of Eating Healthily

In the second paragraph the journal is clearly described as being the Journal of Healthy Eating not the Journal of Eating Healthily. This option is therefore incorrect.

D. Incorrect

69% of individuals are more likely to die if they follow a vegetarian diet

In paragraph three it is stated that individuals who follow a vegetarian diet are 69% less, not more likely, to die. This option is therefore incorrect.

Question 18

We know there are 10 players, the oldest being 16 and the youngest 13. We are also told that there are three times as many 16 year olds as 13 year olds, so there must be at least three 16 year olds and one 13 year old. So if we arrange the ages in order:

16	16	16	a	b	c	d	e	f	13

We know that the modal age is 15 (i.e. the middle value when the data is arranged in order). As we have an even number of data it must lie between b and c. So either b and c are both 15, or b is 16 and c is 14. However we are told that the modal age (most occurring) age is 15 so b and c must be 15, as if they were 16 and 14 then nobody on the team would be 15, and we know this is not true:

16	16	16	a	15	15	d	e	f	13

There can't be any more 16 or 13 year olds, so the rest of the team must be 15 or 14 years old. We are told that there are twice as many 15 year olds as 14 year olds so there must be four 15 year olds (a and d) and two 14 year olds (e and f).

16	16	16	15	15	15	15	14	14	13

Hence the mean age is the sum of the ages ÷ the number of players

$= 149 \div 10$

$= 14.9$

Therefore, the correct answer is C, 14.9

Question 19

The average increase in price between 2007 and 2008.

Cost of oil in 2007 = $60 per barrel; cost in 2008 = $90

Increase in price = $90 − $60 = $30

Increase as a fraction = 30 ÷ 60 = 0.50

Increase as a percentage = 0.50 × 100 = 50%

Therefore the correct answer is B

Question 20

This question can be misleading. At first you might think, that's easy! It's simply the 10% that overlap between credit cards and current accounts. However, there is nothing to tell us that all the 50% of credit card customers do not have current accounts too, with the 10% overlap only having current accounts. This would mean that 50,000 of the customers could in theory have both credit and current accounts. So the correct answer is D.

Question 21

A. Incorrect

The average age of the population is reducing due to mortality

The passage describes that the average age of the population is **increasing** in main due to reduced mortality in the older generation as a result of healthy living. The above statement therefore contradicts the passage and is incorrect.

B. Incorrect

The population dynamics have changed over a 50 year period

The passage describes the change in population dynamics between 1971 to 2005, a difference of 34 years and not a 50 year period. This option is therefore incorrect.

C. **Correct**

The percentage of elderly individuals in the population is increasing as they are living longer

The final sentence in the passage clearly states that the older generation are living longer due to increased healthy living, which accounts for the earlier statement describing an increase in the percentage of over-65s from 13 to 16%. Therefore this statement best describes what is inferred in the passage out of the options available.

D. Incorrect

The number of young people has decreased due to reduced fertility

Although the passage describes that the percentage of under-16s has decreased there is no mention that reduced fertility is the reason, which makes this option incorrect.

Question 22

According to the information provided:

Katie is sitting to the right of Alice with Peter to her left.

Norman is to the left of Angela

Peter is sitting opposite Derek

Derek is sitting next to Katie and Janet

Angela is sitting next to Norman and Peter and opposite Katie

We can therefore determine the following seating plan:

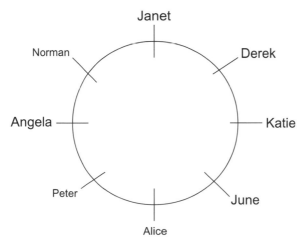

June is therefore sitting next to Alice and Katie. Therefore the correct answer is A.

Question 23

To calculate the average we simply find the sum of the salaries and divide it by the number of people in the group.

So the total of the salaries is: £210,000

We then divide this by 7 which equals £30,000

Therefore the correct answer is C.

Question 24

The options we are given include Louise, John, Peter and James. So we only need to calculate the data for these four people. We need to calculate how much money they earn after tax, and then subsequently how much is left after their monthly outgoings are taken out.

So for Louise: Salary = £21,000, tax at 20% = £4,200

Leaving her with £21,000 − £4,200 = £16,800 after tax per year.

Her monthly take home salary is £16,800 ÷ 12 = £1,400

Her monthly outgoings are £1,500, so she is £100 short each month

For John: Salary = £30,000, tax at 20% = £6,000

Leaving him with £30,000 − £6,000 = £24,000 after tax per year.

His monthly take home salary is £24,000 ÷ 12 = £2,000

His monthly outgoings are £1,800, so he manages to save £200 each month

For Peter: Salary = £25,000, tax at 20% = £5,000

Leaving him with £25,000 − £5,000 = £20,000 after tax per year.

His monthly take home salary is £20,000 ÷ 12 = £1,667

His monthly outgoings are £1,900, so he is £233 short each month

So the answer is B, both Peter and Louise spend more than they earn after tax.

We can just check James to make sure we are correct:

For James: Salary = £42,000, tax at 20% = £8,400

Leaving him with £42,000 − £8,400 = £33,600 after tax per year.

His monthly take home salary is £33,600 ÷ 12 = £2,800

His monthly outgoings are £2,200, so he manages to save £600 each month

Question 25

We are not given any information in the table about how long the staff have worked at the company, so we look for the point which is furthest away from the line of best fit- somebody who earns £30,000. We then use the original table to find who earns this amount of money. The answer is **D**, John. Be careful to read the graph accurately as Kevin earns £31,000, and he is also an option. This question tests your accuracy at graph reading.

Question 26

Louise's salary is £21,000. With a 10% increase it would rise to £21,000 + £2,100 = £23,100 per year.

She is taxed 20% on this, leaving her with £23,100 − £4,620 = £18,480 per year.

Her salary per month = £18,480 ÷ 12 = £1,540 per month.

Her monthly outgoings are £1,500 per month

So she saves £1,540 − £1,500 = £40 a month.

The correct answer is E.

Question 27

1. 2/9 of 126 = 28
2. $28 \times 3\frac{1}{4} = 91$
3. 6/13 of 91 = 42
4. 400% of 42 = 168
5. 5/12 of 168 = 70
6. less 20% of 70 = 56
7. 62.5% of 56 = 35
8. $35 \times 2\frac{1}{7} = 75$
9. 75–39 = 36

Therefore the correct answer is 36

Question 28

A. Incorrect

Firemen are excluded from privileges such as maternity leave and protection against unfair dismissal

There is no reference made to firemen in the passage and this option is therefore incorrect.

B. Incorrect

You can only qualify for maternity leave if you have been employed

The passage clearly states that you can qualify for maternity leave either as an employed or self-employed earner. This option is therefore incorrect.

C. **Correct**

The rules relating to maternity leave do not apply to members of the police force

The passage clearly states that rules relating to maternity leave do not apply for various groups of workers including those who work in the police force. This option is therefore true.

D. Incorrect

All fishermen are entitled to time off for antenatal care

The passage describes that fishermen engaged in share fishing paid solely by how much stock they catch are not entitled to time off for antenatal care. This option is therefore incorrect.

E. Incorrect

All types of company directors are excluded from maternity leave

The passage states that some, but not all, company directors are excluded from maternity leave. This option is therefore incorrect.

Question 29

If we let the standard rate be x and the connection fee be y, we can write the information as two equations:

$6x + y = 2.65$ Equation 1

$15x + y = 5.80$ Equation 2

If we rearrange Equation 1 to make y the subject:

$y = 2.65 - 6x$

We can substitute y into Equation 2:

$15x + 2.65 - 6x = 5.80$

$9x = 5.80 - 2.65$

$9x = 3.15$

$x = 0.35$

We can then substitute x into Equation 1 to find the value of y:

$y = 2.65 - 6x$

$y = 2.65 - (6 \times 0.35)$

$y = 2.65 - 2.10$

$y = 0.55$

So the connection fee is 55p and standard rate per minute 35p

Question 30

A.   50% of 60 = 30 people have a Sunday newspaper delivered, and 60% of 60 = 36 people have a Saturday newspaper delivered. There is an overlap of 6, so at least 6 people must get both delivered.

B.   60 − 36 = 24 people do not have a Saturday newspaper delivered. They may however have a Sunday newspaper delivered, we cannot say whether this is true or not.

C.   30% of 60 = 18 people get a magazine delivered, 36 people get a Sunday newspaper delivered so no more than 18 can have both delivered.

Therefore A and C are both true.

Question 31

A. Incorrect

The Newcastle and Scottish Brewery have made a loss of 19% compared to last year's net profits

Although the passage states that the Newcastle and Scottish Brewery net profits are down by 9% in the first six months it cannot be concluded that a loss of 19% has been made in the last year. This option therefore incorrectly describes the main conclusion of the passage.

B. Incorrect

The reason targets have been reached by Newcastle and Scottish Brewery is due in part to there being a Rugby World Cup

Although the passage describes the lack of Rugby World Cup as a reason for affecting the targets it clearly states the targets have **not** been reached. This option states that the targets **have** been reached due to the Rugby World Cup which contradicts the passage. This option is therefore incorrect.

C. Incorrect

An upturn in the weather will ensure that Newcastle and Scottish Brewery hit their target

Although this statement may go some way to best describing the passage, it is somewhat ambiguous and does not describe the passage as a whole and when compared to Option D is the lesser of the two options which best summarises the passage.

D. Correct

It is unlikely that Newcastle and Scottish Brewery will hit their targets this year

This statement best summarises the passage as a whole relating to the fact that it is unlikely that the brewery will hit their targets this year.

E. Incorrect

Bad weather in the US has caused a loss in revenue for Newcastle and Scottish Brewery

The passage does not describe the state of the weather in the US and this statement does not best summarise the passage.

Question 32

In the first 20 minutes she rowed 6,000m

Between 20 and 40 minutes she rowed 5% less than 6,000m, 5% of 6,000 = 300 therefore she rowed 6,000 − 300 = 5,700m

Between 40 and 60 minutes she rowed 10% further than she did between 20 and 40 minutes 10% of 5,700 = 570, therefore she rowed 5,700 + 570 = 6,270m

She therefore rowed 6,270 − 6,000 = 270m more in the final 20 minutes compared to the first 20 minutes.

This expressed as a percentage = (270 ÷ 6,000) × 100 = 27/6% = 4.5%

Therefore the correct answer is D, 4.5%

Question 33

A. *The distance travelled between 0 and 10 minutes is half that travelled between 30 and 40 minutes.*

This is true; distance travelled is calculated by the area under the graph.

B. *The lorry was travelling twice as quickly during 30–40 minutes as during 0–10 minutes.*

This is false, the average speed between 0–10 minutes may be half of that between 30–40, but as the lorry's speed during the first 10 minutes was not constant this statement is not true.

C. *The average speed between 30 and 40 minutes is twice that of the average speed between 0 and 10 minutes.*

This statement is true. The average speed of the lorry during 0–10 minutes was 30mph, and the average speed during 30–40 minutes was 60mph.

D. *The lorry travelled quicker during the first 10 minutes than it did during 30–40 minutes of its journey.*

This statement is false. The lorry was not travelling quicker in the first 10 minutes, it was accelerating but it only reached a top speed of 60 mph, which is the speed the lorry was travelling at during 30–40 minutes of its journey.

The correct answers are therefore A and C.

Question 34

The first digit we know is 2

The third digit is directly below the second; all possibilities are:

$2 + 1 + 4$

$2 + 3 + 6$

$2 + 4 + 7$

$2 + 5 + 8$

$2 + 6 + 9$

$2 + 8 + 0$

The fourth digit plus the first digit (2) is the same as the third digit. (So the fourth digit = third digit minus 2)

$2 + 1 + 4 + 2$ not possible as 2 appears twice

$2 + 3 + 6 + 4$

$2 + 4 + 7 + 5$

$2 + 5 + 8 + 6$

$2 + 6 + 9 + 7$

$2 + 8 + 0 + (-2)$ not possible as negative numbers not allowed.

We know the total of the digits is 29 so we can calculate the fifth digit:

$2 + 3 + 6 + 4 = 15$ (29–15 = 14) not possible

$2 + 4 + 7 + 5 = 18$ (29–18 =11) not possible

$2 + 5 + 8 + 6 = 21$ (29–21 =8). 8 already appears in the code so is not possible

$2 + 6 + 9 + 7 = 24$ (29–24 = 5) only possible answer.

The correct code is $2 + 6 + 9 + 7 + 5$

Therefore the correct answer is C, 5.

Question 35

The key to answering the question is to establish the facts relating to the answer options provided which relate to either the venue, day/time of visiting or activity. A simple table helps to clarify these facts

Venue	James	Joe	John
AbsGym	Gym 7 days a week	Swims Sat and Sun	Gym Sun to Thurs 9am–4pm
ProBowl	Bowling Weds and Fri	Bowling Monday	Pool Saturday
Riversmeet Leisure Centre	Swims Sunday	Spinning classes, Mon, Weds and Fri	Spinning classes Weds

Using the above information

A. Incorrect

They are all attending spinning classes

According to the passage only Joe and John attend spinning classes therefore this option is incorrect as it excludes James.

B. Correct

It is a Sunday

This is the correct answer. They must be present at the AbsGym changing room as James visits seven days a week, Joe swims there on a Sunday and John uses the gym on a Sunday.

C. Incorrect

They must be at the Riversmeet Leisure Centre

According to the passage at most there are only ever two of the individuals, Joe and John, present together which is on a Wednesday.

D. Incorrect

The time must be 9.30pm

Although the passage does not state the time that James and Joe visit the various facilities it does state that John has a student membership. This restricts his use to between the hours of 9am and 4pm which makes this option highly unlikely and therefore incorrect.

E. Incorrect

It is a Saturday

Although James and Joe visit the AbsGym on a Saturday the passage clearly states that John only attends the Absgym on a Sunday which therefore rules out this option as the correct answer.

Mock Exam Paper Answers: Section 2

Question 1

(i)   The chemical that neutralizes stomach acid is (B) bile, which is produced in the liver and stored in the gall bladder. It is an alkali and is also responsible for emulsifying fats.

(ii) The enzyme which breaks down proteins into amino acids is protease (C). This is secreted in the stomach, pancreas and small intestine.

(iii) Amylase is a carbohydrase (A). It is produced in the salivary glands and breaks down starch into sugar.

(iv) Lipase (D) catalyses the hydrolysis (breakdown) of triglycerides (fats) into fatty acids and glycerol. It is secreted by the pancreas and small intestine.

Question 2

There is a total of 12 gums in the packet.

The probability of getting two the same colour

$$= P(\text{red} \times \text{red}) + P(\text{black} \times \text{black}) + P(\text{green} \times \text{green})$$
$$= (3/12 \times 2/11) + (4/12 \times 3/11) + (5/12 \times 4/11)$$
$$= 6/132 + 12/132 + 20/132$$
$$= 38/132$$
$$= 19/66$$

We always present fractions in their lowest form, so the correct answer is **B**.

The important thing to remember here is that after one sweet is picked there is one less of this colour and one less in total, so the probability of picking another sweet the same colour is reduced.

Question 3

The mass is the number of protons and neutrons. The atomic number is the number of protons.

We are told that an isotope has the same number of protons but differing neutrons. Therefore the atomic number stays the same: 6, but the mass increases.

The only option that fits both criteria is D.

Question 4

Temperature receptors in the hand detect an increase in temperature, the receptors activate a signalling cascade which is transmitted to the spinal cord via a sensory neuron (as it is a simple, involuntary reflex and does not need to go via the brain).

An impulse is transmitted to the muscles in the arm via a motor neuron resulting in the removal of the hand from the hot water.

The correct order of events is D, B, E, C, A

Question 5

$V = \frac{1}{3} \pi r^2 h$

$3V = \pi r^2 h$ (multiply both sides by 3)

$r^2 = 3V/\pi h$ (divide both sides by πh)

$r = \sqrt{(3V/\pi h)}$ (square root both sides)

Question 6

A. Correct

Both sodium and potassium are important ions in controlling blood pressure

B. Incorrect

The kidneys do not release ADH, this is released by the pituitary gland, and controls the levels of water the kidneys reabsorb

C. Incorrect

The removal of waste products from the body does not directly affect blood pressure

D. Correct

The amount of water reabsorbed affects the volume of the blood. An increase in blood volume results in an increase in blood pressure

E. Incorrect

Simply removing potassium is not how the kidneys maintain blood pressure. Yes, the kidneys do control the amount of potassium reabsorbed – however the statement 'removing' is too vague

So the correct answers are A and D.

Question 7

We are given the equation to calculate the momentum of the bullet:

Change in momentum = $mv - mu$

We know the mass of the bullet to be 50g = 0.05kg, and the initial velocity of the bullet to be 0

So the change in momentum = 0.05v

We can substitute this into the second equation:

Force (N) = change in momentum (kg m/s) ÷ Time (s)

Force (N) = 0.05v (kg m/s) ÷ Time (s)

5,000 = 0.05v ÷ 0.01

making v the subject

0.05v = 5,000 × 0.01

0.05v = 50

v = 1000 m/s

Therefore the answer is A, 1,000 m/s

Question 8

$\overrightarrow{XY} = \overrightarrow{XO} + \overrightarrow{OA} + \overrightarrow{AY}$

= −2/3b + a + (1/2 b-a)

= −2/3b + a + 1/2b − 1/2a

= −4/6b + a + 3/6b −1/2a

= −1/6b + 1/2a

Therefore the correct answer is C, −1/6b + 1/2a

Question 9

To calculate the energy change, we need to calculate the energy taken to break the bonds of the reactants, and the energy required to form the bonds of the products.

Reactants: CH_4 = 4 C-H bonds = 4×400 = 1600

$2O_2$ = 2 0=0 bonds = 2×500 = 1000

So the energy required to break the bonds of the reactants is 2,600kJ

Products: CO_2 = 2 C=0 bonds = 2×800 = 1600

$2H_2O$ = 4 0-H bonds = 4×450 = 1800

So the energy released when the bonds of the reactants are formed is 3,400kJ

So the overall energy change is −2,600 (the value is negative as energy is required to break bonds) + 3,400 = 800kJ (heat is given out so the reaction is exothermic).

The correct answer is A.

Question 10

Both 3 and 4 must be carriers of the faulty gene, as their daughter inherited two faulty copies of the gene and suffers with cystic fibrosis. 6 must also be a carrier as 6's son would definitely inherit one faulty gene from his affected mother, and as he has cystic fibrosis must have inherited another from his father (6). 6 must have inherited his faulty gene from one of his parents – so either 1 or 2 must be carriers. We do not have enough information to say whether 5, 7 and 8 are carriers or not.

Therefore the correct answer is **E**, either 1 or 2 are carriers and 3 + 4 + 6 are all carriers.

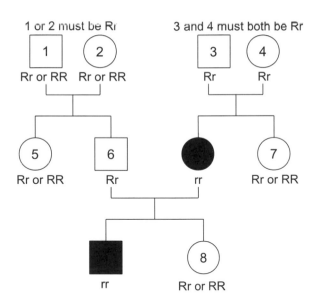

Question 11

The area of the square = $(2\sqrt{5} + \sqrt{3})(2\sqrt{5} + \sqrt{3})$

Expanding out the brackets:

$(2\sqrt{5} \times 2\sqrt{5}) + (\sqrt{3} \times \sqrt{3}) + (\sqrt{3} \times 2\sqrt{5}) + (2\sqrt{5} \times \sqrt{3})$

Simplifying the above:

$4\sqrt{25} + \sqrt{9} + 2\sqrt{15} + 2\sqrt{15}$
$= (4 \times 5) + 3 + 4\sqrt{15}$
$= 23 + 4\sqrt{15}$ cm^2

Therefore the correct answer is B.

Question 12

The equation we need here is $F = m \times a$

First we need to calculate the acceleration. Using the following formula:

$$\text{Acceleration} = \frac{\text{change in velocity}}{\text{time}}$$

$= 5/7$ m/s^2

We can then use the first equation to find the force:

$F = m \times a$
$= 700 \times 5/7$
$= 500$N

Therefore the answer is C.

Question 13

Oxygenated blood from the lungs enters the heart via the pulmonary vein (14). It enters into the left atrium (5). It then passes through the mitral value (11) into the left ventricle (4); from here it is pumped through the aortic valve (10), to the aorta (1) and then on to the rest of the body.

The correct answer is therefore A.

Question 14

A force of 5N is applied to an area of 0.1m² in the master cylinder. We need to calculate the pressure this transmits to the slave cylinder.

Pressure (N/m^2) = Force (N) ÷ area (m²)

= 5 ÷ 0.1

= 50 N/ m²

So a pressure of 50 N/m² is transmitted to the piston in the slave cylinder:

Force = pressure x area

= 50 × 2

=100N

Therefore a force of 100N is applied to the brake pad.

Question 15

We can take π to equal 3

A is a hemisphere

$$
\begin{aligned}
\text{Volume of sphere} \quad &= 4/3 \; \pi \; r^3 \\
&= 4/3 \times 3 \times 4^3 \\
&= 4^4 \\
&= 256 \; \text{cm}^3
\end{aligned}
$$

So volume of hemisphere $= 256/2 = 128 \; \text{cm}^3$

B is a cone

$$
\begin{aligned}
\text{Volume of cone} \quad &= \tfrac{1}{3} \; \pi \; r^2 h \\
&= \tfrac{1}{3} \times 3 \; (4^2 \times 4) \\
&= 4^3 \\
&= 64 \; \text{cm}^3
\end{aligned}
$$

C is a cylinder

$$
\begin{aligned}
\text{Volume of cylinder} \quad &= \pi \; r^2 h \\
&= 3 \; (4^2 \times 4) \\
&= 192 \; \text{cm}^3
\end{aligned}
$$

Therefore

C has a greater volume than A, and A has a greater volume than B. So C has a greater volume than B. So **B** is correct.

Also A has a volume less than that of C but greater than that of B. So **E** is correct.

A.   A does have a greater volume than B, but B is not greater than C so this is false

C.   B does not have a greater volume than A so this is false

D.   C does have a volume greater than A but it is not less than B so this is false

Therefore the correct answers are B and E

Question 16

To calculate the distance from a velocity (or speed) time graph we simply need to calculate the area under the graph. In this question, it can be done by breaking the area into three sections.

Section 1: From 0 to 20m/s in 10 seconds (a triangle)

Section 2: A constant velocity of 20m/s from 10–30 seconds (a rectangle)

Section 3: From 20 m/s to 0 from 30 to 60 seconds (a triangle)

Section 1: Area of triangle
$$= \frac{1}{2} \text{ base} \times \text{height}$$
$$= \frac{1}{2} \ 10 \times 20$$
$$= 5 \times 20$$
$$= 100\text{m}$$

Section 2: Area of rectangle
$$= \text{base} \times \text{height}$$
$$= (30{-}10) \times 20$$
$$= 20 \times 20$$
$$= 400\text{m}$$

Section 3: Area of triangle
$$= \frac{1}{2} \text{ base} \times \text{height}$$
$$= \frac{1}{2} \ (60 - 30) \times 20$$
$$= \frac{1}{2} \ 30 \times 20$$
$$= 300\text{m}$$

Therefore the total distance travelled is 100 + 400 + 300m = 800m.

The correct answer is therefore D.

Question 17

The true answers are A, B, and E.

C. They may work quicker at higher temperature, but the question does not state what the temperature is, so this is not correct as temperatures above 37°C may cause the enzyme to denature, and not work so efficiently.

D. Activation energy is the energy which must be overcome to get a reaction started. Enzymes lower the activation energy by either positioning the substrates so they are in an optimal position to react, or by breaking covalent bonds.

Question 18

$Fe_2O_3 + 2Al \longrightarrow 2Fe + Al_2O_3$

M_r (Relative molecular mass) of $Fe_2O_3 = (56 \times 2) + (16 \times 3)$ = 160

A_r (Atomic mass) of $Fe = 2 \times 56 = 112$

Moles reacted = 40/160 = ¼

So ¼ of a mole of Fe_2O_3 was used in the reaction. This would yield $112 \times ¼ = 28g$ of iron.

The correct answer is therefore 28g

Question 19

Smoking greatly increases the chance of developing Coronary Heart Disease (CHD); the main reasons for this are that:

A. True

It causes increased blood cholesterol and blood pressure, which causes fat to be deposited in the blood vessels (atheromas), resulting in the narrowing of the blood vessels which increases the risk of heart attacks and strokes.

B. False

Nicotine causes constriction of the blood vessels; it does not directly stop the heart from working properly.

C. True

Carbon monoxide reduces the affinity haemoglobin has for oxygen, therefore reducing the amount of oxygen the red blood cells can transport. This reduces the amount of oxygen delivered to the vital organs which can increase the risk of CHD.

D. False

Lack of exercise is a risk factor for CHD, but this is irrespective of whether you smoke or not. Smoking does not make you less likely to exercise.

E. False

Tar does not build up in the arteries; it builds up in the lungs when cigarette smoke is inhaled.

The correct answers are therefore A and C.

Question 20

A half life is defined as the time taken for the radioactive count rate of a substance to fall by half of its starting level.

The easiest way to calculate this it to take a value on the Y axis and find the corresponding time on the X axis.

e.g. Time at 250 counts = 7 days,

The activity at 0 days = 500 c/s.

activity at 7 days = 250 c/s.

The activity has halved (500 to 250 c/s) in 7 days.

Therefore the answer is C, the half life of the substance is 7 days.

Question 21

$$aI_2 + bNa_2S_2O_3 \longrightarrow cNaI + dNa_2S_4O_6$$

If we start with b, we have 2S's and 3O's on the left and 4S's and 6O's on the right. If we make b 2, and d 1, then that means the O's and S's balance, but we have 2 extra Na's on the right. If we make c 2, that makes the Na's balance and gives us 2I's on the right which if a is 1 we have on the left, so

$a = 1, b = 2, c = 2, d = 1$.

Question 22

Insulin is released when the blood sugar level is high; it causes excess glucose to be converted to glycogen which is stored in the liver. When blood sugar levels are low, glucagon is released which converts glycogen to glucose.

Therefore the correct answer is A.

Question 23

The voltage and turns across the coils are related by the following equation:

$$\frac{\text{Voltage across primary}}{\text{Voltage across secondary}} = \frac{\text{number of turns on primary}}{\text{number of turns on secondary}}$$

$$\frac{Vp}{Vs} = \frac{Np}{Ns}$$

Substituting the values we know into the equation:

$$\frac{230V}{Vs} = \frac{1000}{100}$$

$$Vs = \frac{230 \times 100}{1000}$$

$$Vs = 23V$$

The voltage across the secondary coil is 23V

Question 24

A. Repopulation of endangered species – Yes, populations of endangered species could be cloned to prevent extinction

B. Creating genetically modified crops – Yes, this is currently in process, e.g. growing disease-resistant crops

C. Asexual reproduction – Yes, this is a form of cloning e.g. in plants, as each time a plant reproduces asexually its offspring is an identical copy

D. Generating new tissues and organs for transplants – Yes, new organs can be grown from either stem cells or in another organism

E. IVF – No, IVF is In Vitro Fertilisation, where an egg is fertilised by a sperm in a laboratory environment and inserted into the womb. The process does not involve cloning.

The correct answer is therefore E.

Question 25

$$1 - \frac{(3x+7)}{2} = \frac{(x+4)}{4}$$

Step 1: Multiply both sides by 2:

$$2 - \frac{2(3x+7)}{2} = \frac{2(x+4)}{4}$$

Step 2: Expand out bracket

$$2 - 3x + 7 = \frac{(x+4)}{2}$$

$$9 - 3x = \frac{(x+4)}{2}$$

Step 3: Multiply both sides by 2:

$$18 - 6x = x + 4$$

Step 4: $+ 6x$ both sides

$$18 = 7x + 4$$

Step 5: -4 both sides

$$14 = 7x$$

Step 6: divide both sides by 7

$$x = 2$$

The correct answer is therefore 2.

Question 26

Mitosis is the process by which asexual reproduction occurs.

1. The chromosomes condense and become visible
2. The nuclear envelope disappears
3. Chromosomes move to the equator of the spindle
4. The chromatids separate
5. The cytoplasm divides

The correct order is E, D, C, B, A

Question 27

In Graph 1, the solid line has a greater gradient than the control. This means that it has a higher resistance than the control as the current is able to flow less freely since:

Resistance = voltage ÷ current.

We can check this by calculating the gradient (i.e. resistance) at a point, at a voltage of 0.1V, the control wire has a current of 1A, a resistance of $0.1 \div 1 = 0.10$ohms. At the same voltage the unknown component/wire has a current of 0.5A, and a resistance of $0.1 \div 0.5 = 0.2$ohms.

An increase in resistance can be due to the presence of a resistor or due to a decreased wire thickness, increased wire length or an increase in temperature. In this case as it's the only option which could be correct, it is an increase in temperature which causes the higher resistance, and hence the steeper line on the graph.

In Graph 2, the solid line represents the presence of a filament lamp. A cold bulb has a lower resistance and draws more current. This causes it to increase in temperature which leads to an increase in resistance. This is why the gradient of the line increases with increasing voltage.

In Graph 3 the solid line represents a diode, as these allow only a tiny flow of current at low voltages. Once the voltage is increased above a certain level the diode switches on and allows current to flow.

In Graph 4, the solid line exhibits a smaller gradient than the control wire. This means that it has a lower resistance than the control as:

Resistance = voltage ÷ current.

We can check this by calculating the gradient at a point. At a voltage of 0.05V, the control has a current of 0.5A, and a resistance of 0.05 ÷ 0.5 = 0.1ohms. At the same voltage the test unknown has a current of 1A, a resistance of 0.05 ÷ 1.0 = 0.05 ohms.

A decrease in resistance can be due to a change in the metal used in the wire, a decrease in the length of the wire, or a decrease in temperature. From the options we are given, it must be due to a decreased wire length.

The correct answer is therefore D.

Mock Exam Paper Answers: Section 3

1   'Body and soul cannot be separated for purposes of treatment, for they are one and indivisible. Sick minds must be healed as well as sick bodies'.
(C. Jeff Miller)

What do you understand this statement to mean?

Present examples to illustrate where conditions of mind and body are directly connected, and where they must be dealt with separately

How would you propose the conflict between the treatment of physical and psychological illnesses be resolved?

Possible Answer

One could say this statement refers to the way that the mind and body are inextricably linked, and should be treated as such during most medical treatments. It could be argued that the majority of serious illnesses affect both the body and the mind, and that this should be considered when the clinician is choosing the best course of treatment. For example, Huntington's disease affects the patient physically through involuntary muscle movements, as well as psychologically through depression, mood swings and memory loss.

In many cases, physical symptoms are related to a mental condition. For example, a patient suffering from severe anxiety may experience heart palpitations and chest pain. Treatment should focus on the mental issue – the anxiety – as this is the cause of the physical symptoms. Equally, the opposite can be true – physical conditions may cause mental problems. An example of this would be a patient suffering from sexual dysfunction who develops depression as a result. In such cases, it is the clinician's job to decide which constitutes the cause and which constitutes the effect, for a common symptom of depression is sexual dysfunction. This is where the skill and experience of the clinician becomes paramount to a successful diagnosis and course of treatment. There are times when both physical and psychological treatments are necessary. Treatment of an alcoholic might require medication to reduce the symptoms of withdrawal, while additional medication or counselling may be needed to deal with the psychological causes and effects of the illness. There are, however, instances when the mind and body must be treated separately. An example would be in the treatment of a cancer patient. The focus has to be on the treatment of the cancer itself, the physical problem rather than any mental problems which may arise in the patient due to the trauma of having a life-threatening illness.

It is possible that the conflict between the treatment of physical and psychological illnesses could be somewhat solved by embracing a more holistic approach. Increasingly, mainstream healthcare professionals are taking on board holistic theories, such as the idea that health is not just an absence of biological faults but more an all-encompassing wellbeing of body and soul. This is possibly the way forward for modern medicine.

2　'A little knowledge that acts is worth infinitely more than much knowledge that is idle'.
　(Kahlil Gibran)

　What do you think the above statement implies?

　Demonstrate through examples where acting on a small amount of knowledge may be less helpful than not acting on a wealth of knowledge

To what extent should a clinician prioritise action over investigation?

Possible Answer

It could be argued that instinct is our greatest natural defence against potential threats. Acting quickly, with little or no real knowledge of a situation, could potentially mean the difference between life and death; conversely, refusal to act for any reason – regardless of whether the individual involved is capable of managing the situation – could result in unnecessary delay and even permanent damage or death. Knowing when to react instantly and when to assess the situation before making a decision are essential skills for any medical practitioner.

Any trauma doctor or paramedic needs to have the ability to react quickly to a situation while under pressure and usually with relatively little information to work with. The skill of a paramedic is to make the correct decision under such circumstances, but he or she would be calling on past knowledge and experience, combined with their natural instincts. A passer-by at the same accident scene may possess that same instinct to help others – the difference would be that the average passer-by would not be equipped with the same medical knowledge. Having watched a medical drama or documentary the night before, the passer-by may determine that the victim is suffocating and in need of a tracheotomy; realising that time is short, the passer-by may decide that, instead of calling for appropriate help and waiting for a medical professional, they need to act on the spot and perform the procedure themselves. They may be lucky; more likely, however, is that they could puncture a vein or artery, perforate the vocal cords, or pierce the oesophagus. Where the victim may have survived long enough to receive help, they would now bleed or choke to death before professional help could arrive.

A clinician should always investigate as far as possible for any patient, but a lengthy diagnosis is not always possible and fast action will inevitably be required. The true danger lies in those acting on perceived knowledge or in a situation well beyond their capabilities. Acting on the smallest amount of knowledge with no real comprehension of how it may relate to differing circumstances can only be dangerous, and unless the patient is certainly facing death either way, waiting for the necessary help is always the best course of action.

3   'A person cannot know more than they have experienced; without experience, a person cannot understand that which they know.'

Explain in your own words what this statement suggests

Give examples of how different levels of knowledge and experience, or lack thereof, could affect patient care

How far do you believe that knowledge and experience are dependent on one another?

Possible Answer

Confusing knowledge and experience is potentially a very dangerous thing for any medical professional to do, and though the two concepts are inextricably linked, they cannot be simply interchanged. Knowledge could be defined as the possession of information which ultimately leads to the ability to perform an action, whilst experience could be defined as practice in performing those actions; knowledge, therefore, tells us *what* to do, whilst experience tells us *how*, and provides a full understanding of the implications and applications of the knowledge we possess.

Within a clinical setting, lack of knowledge or experience could lead to failures in patient care. A medical student, for example, must be expected to possess a certain level of knowledge, but cannot yet call on experience; they must rely on the experience of more senior doctors to ensure that their knowledge is applied safely and correctly. A trainee surgeon, regardless of how much they know, could not be expected to perform complex heart surgery with no experience. Even if they knew exactly what to do, lack of experience would render them unable to handle unexpected complications; thus, lack of experience leads to a lack of adaptability, an essential skill for doctors under pressured circumstances. Performing such an operation without any real understanding or insight would ultimately endanger a patient and potentially lead to death. Whilst knowledge is finite and potentially has limits, experience is both abstract and unlimited; knowledge can be lost or forgotten much more easily than experience. Experience can also be sought through failure, particularly where knowledge may be incomplete.

Based on this argument, it is certainly safe to assume that knowledge and experience are symbiotic. It seems sensible to suggest that experience can improve knowledge through enabling a hands-on learning approach; though core knowledge is ultimately vital, it is only through experience that we can learn how important that knowledge is. As a doctor, experience is vital; within real-world situations knowledge cannot be relied upon in isolation, and must be tempered by experience to ensure safe and effective practice.

Chapter 8 Conclusion

By reading through our examples and working through our mock test, you should now have an understanding of not just what to expect from the BMAT, but how to prepare for the exam itself. The most important things to remember are:

Preparation

It can't be stressed enough that preparation is the key to success in the BMAT; if you turn up on the day without conducting any preparation, the chances are you won't perform as well as someone who's spent time refreshing their knowledge and skills and getting into the correct frame of mind. Remember – it's more about how you answer the questions than how much you know.

Start early

Don't leave it until the night before the exam to start reading the British Medical Journal or sifting through past papers. The BMAT isn't a test you can cram for; you need time to absorb the knowledge and prepare your mind for the questions you will be facing. Start your preparation as early as you can and make sure you set out a plan – you won't get anywhere learning random facts and figures, so set yourself a timetable and build up your studies until the exam itself.

Don't panic

You'll be under pressure in the exam and you'll have to manage your time carefully, so the key is to stay calm. If you don't know the answer, move on. Don't waste valuable time forcing yourself to answer a question if you can't work it out. This is likely to lead to frustration and could end up with you running out of time before you get to the questions you *can* answer. Never leave any question unanswered, even if you guess; you still have a chance of selecting the right answer. You have nothing to lose as you will not be penalised for a wrong answer.

The aim of this book has been to provide you with an insight into the BMAT and give you the opportunity to practise the various questions you will come up against. Our hope is that by following the principles and steps contained in this book you will be able to confidently complete your BMAT with excellent results.

If you feel that you still require further practice and would like to experience the BMAT in an online format, you can subscribe to our online revision lessons at www.developmedica.com.

In addition to this book, the Developmedica website (www.developmedica.com) contain lots of free resources, including details of 'hot topics' in the medical and dental world, to help you prepare for your application to medical or dental school and subsequent interview.

We strongly recommend that you do seek more information from the universities to which you are applying, and also from the official BMAT websites, to ensure that you are fully prepared for your BMAT.

From all at Developmedica, we would like to wish you every success in securing your place at university.

Good Luck!

More titles in the Entry to Medical School Series

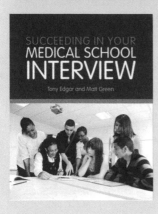

September 2009

148 pages

Paperback

978-0-9556746-4-8

An essential student resource which looks at the part the Medical School Interview plays in the overall process through which students are selected to study Medicine, and will help school leavers, mature and graduate students alike.

In this book Tony Edgar and Matt Green:

- Look at the part the Medical School Interview plays in the overall process through which students are selected to study Medicine

- Describe the criteria against which interview panels conduct their assessments

- Highlight the importance of thorough preparation in advance of the interview

- Use topical examples to illustrate the key principles underpinning the successful performance on the day

- Provide tips on what to do and what not to do

Most importantly of all, this engaging, easy to use and comprehensive guide will help you give your very best account of yourself in your own unique way.

develop medica

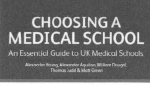
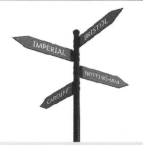

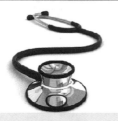

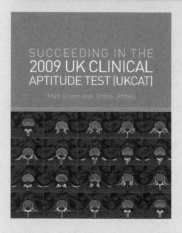

More titles in the Entry to Medical School Series

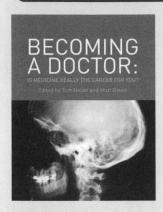

January 2009

152 pages

Paperback

978-0-9556746-6-2

develop
medica

www.developmedica.com

More titles in the Entry to Medical School Series

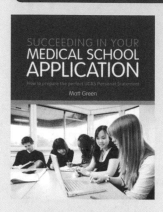

As the competition for Medical School places continues to increase, it is more important than ever to ensure that your application reflects what the admissions tutors will be looking for. This book will help school leavers, graduates and mature individuals applying to medical school, together with parents and teachers, to make their UCAS Personal Statement both compelling and convincing reading. In this book, Matt Green:

- Describes the context of the Medical School Personal Statement within the application process

- Highlights the fact that selection for Medical School implies selection for the medical profession

- Sets out the essential contents of the Medical Personal Statement, the key steps in its preparation and what to include and what not to include

- Drafts and refines a fictitious UCAS Personal Statement, making for a most valuable case study through which the consideration of all the important, key principles are brought to life

- New to this edition - Includes 30 high quality Medical Personal Statement examples to provide inspiration during the writing process

March 2009

120 pages

Paperback

978-1-906839-05-5

£14.99

By using this engaging, easy to use and comprehensive book, you can remove so much of the uncertainty surrounding your Medical School application.

develop
medica

www.developmedica.com